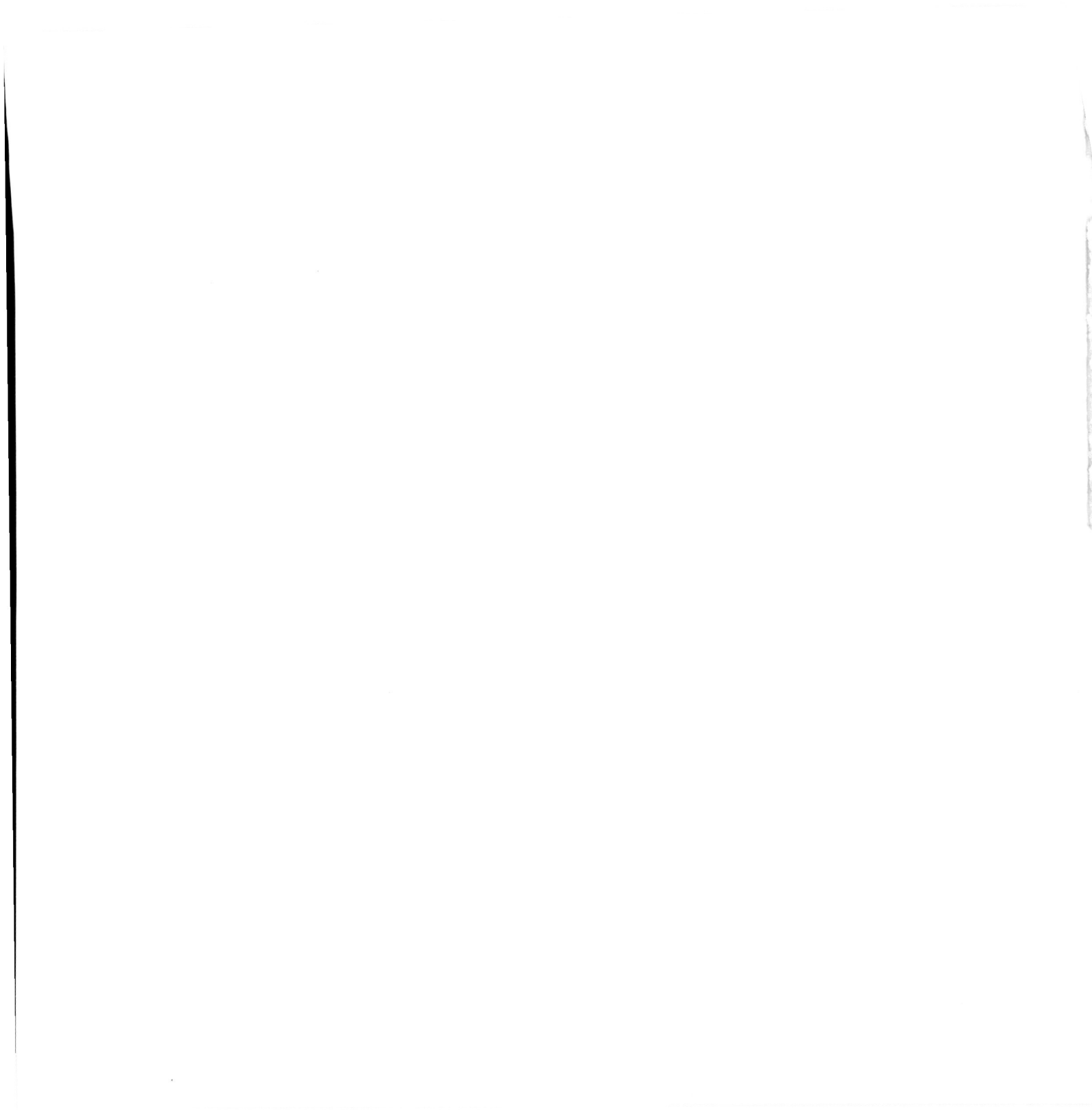

BONK!
and
what's
next.

Written and Illustrated by
Doug Rucker
Layout by Helane Freeman

Doug Rucker
Vilimapubco
Malibu, CA
ruckerdoug@gmail.com

For permission requests, sales to U.S. bookstores and wholesalers, or to inquire about quantity discounts, please contact the publisher at the email address above.
Printed in the United States of America

Library of Congress Control Number: 2018900305

ISBN 978-0-9996811-0-7

First Edition
10 9 8 7 6 5 4 3 2 1

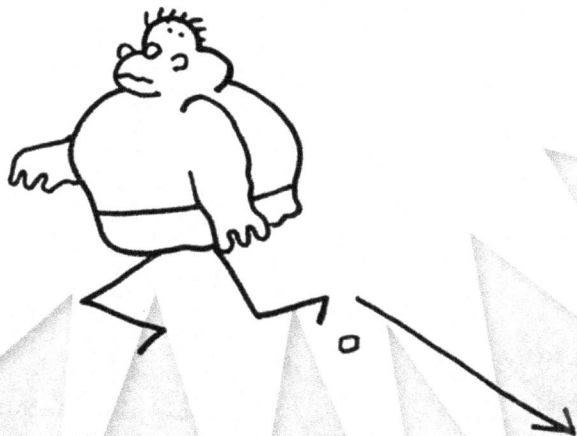

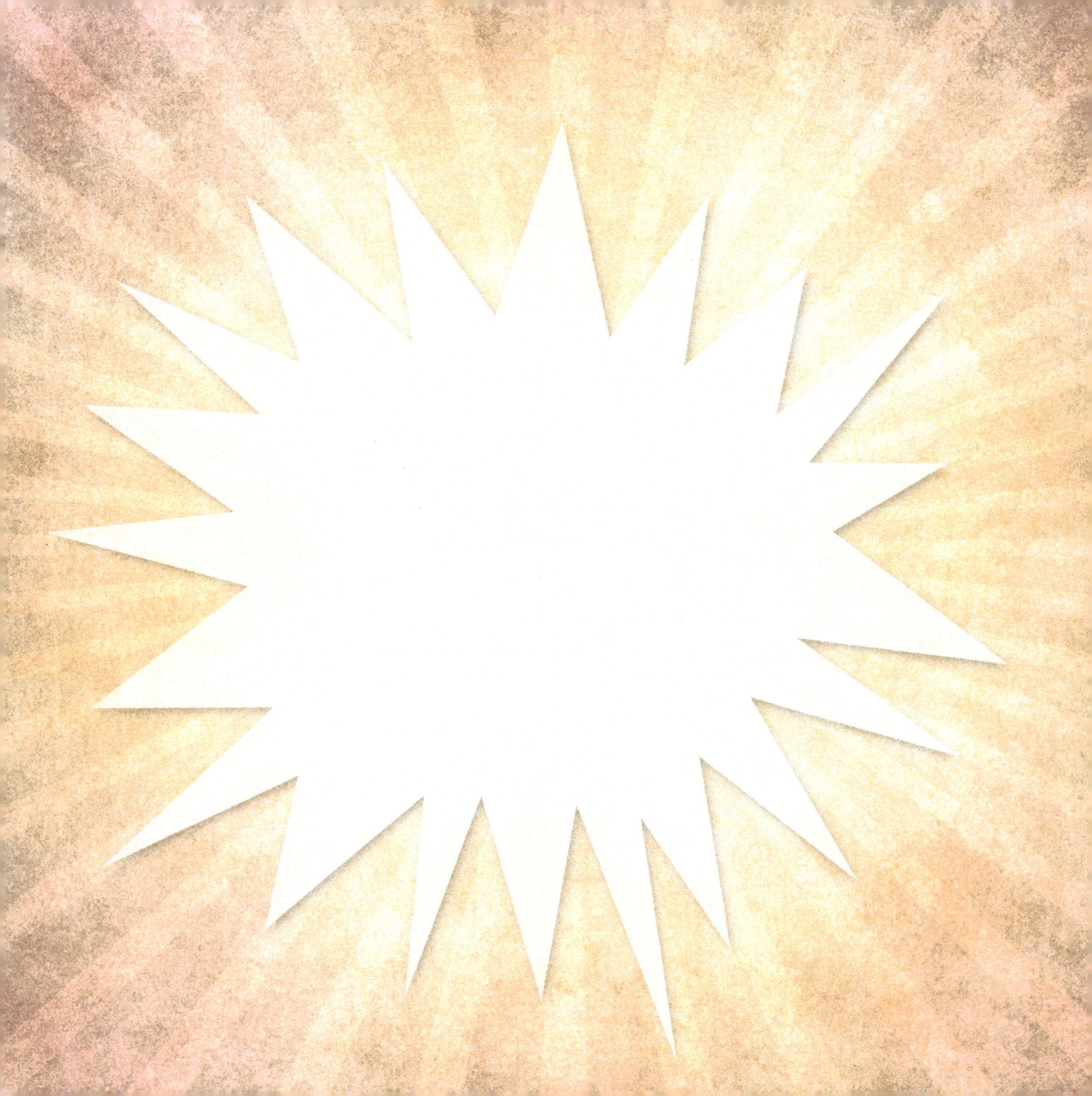

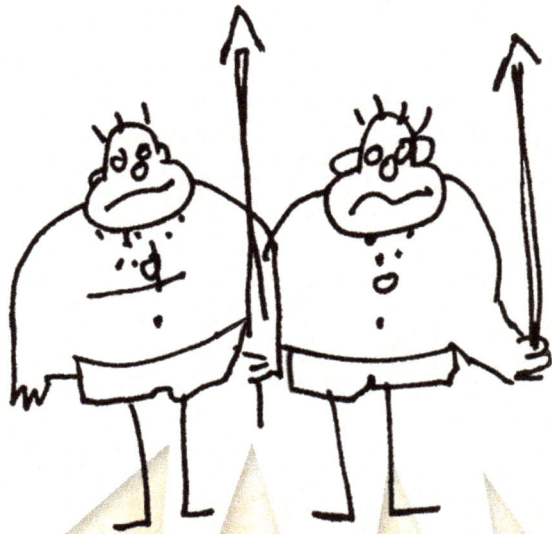

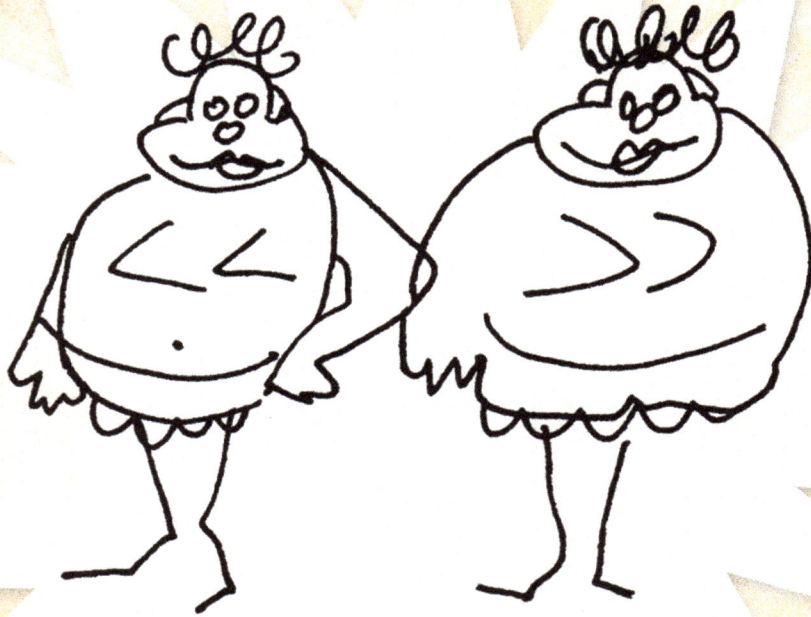

then, women

then, children.

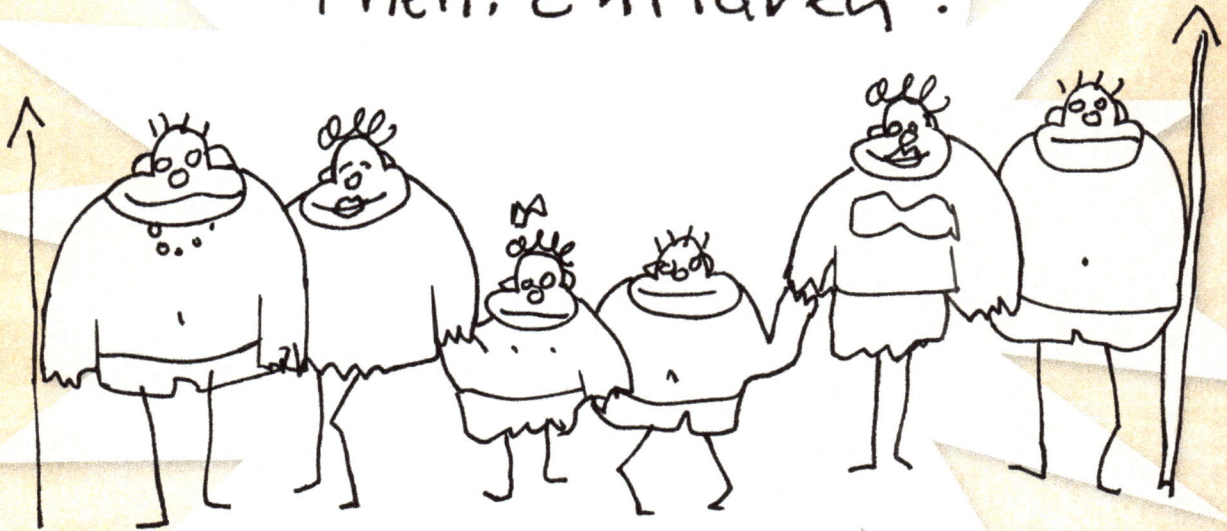

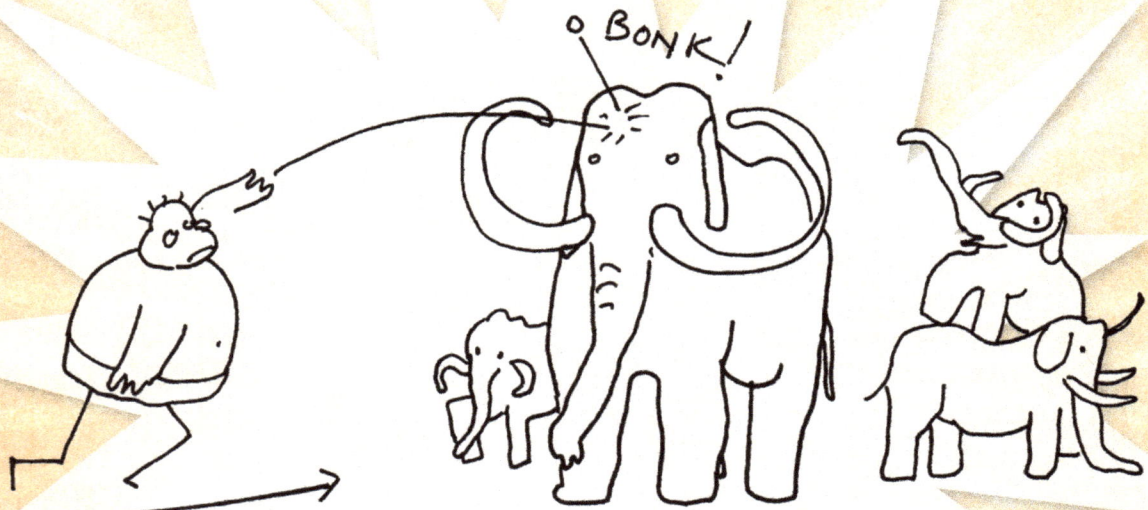

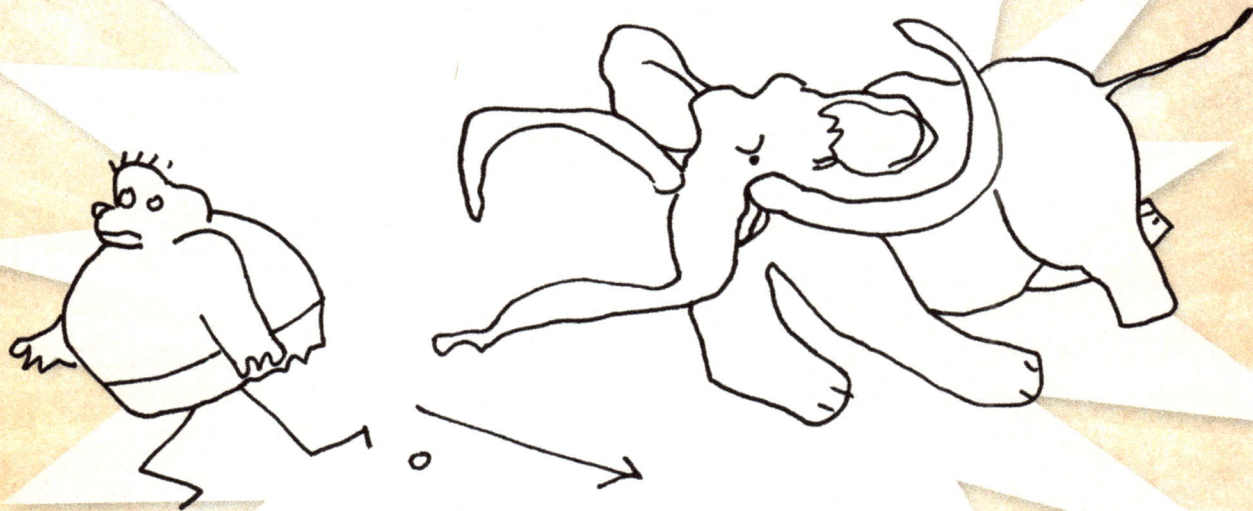

it wasn't always easy.

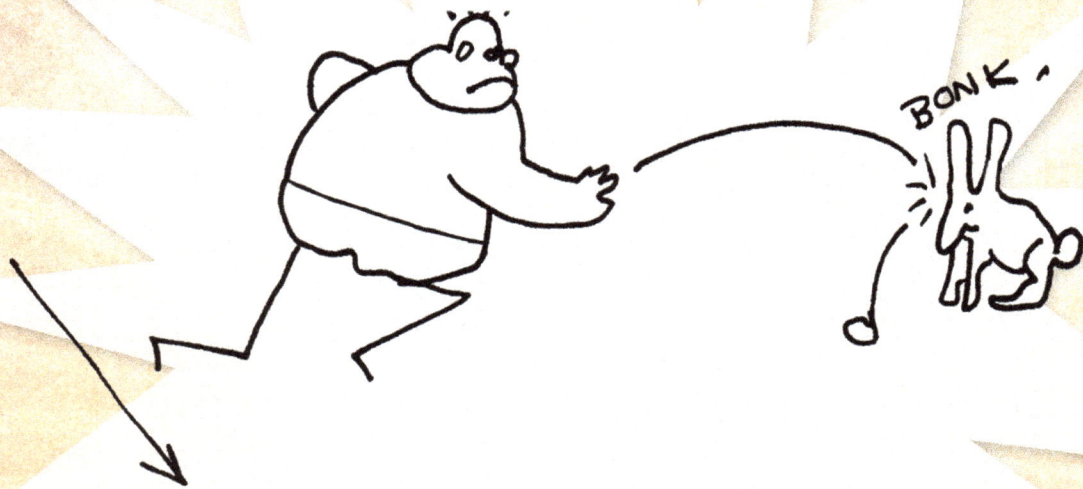

First man hunted jackrabbits

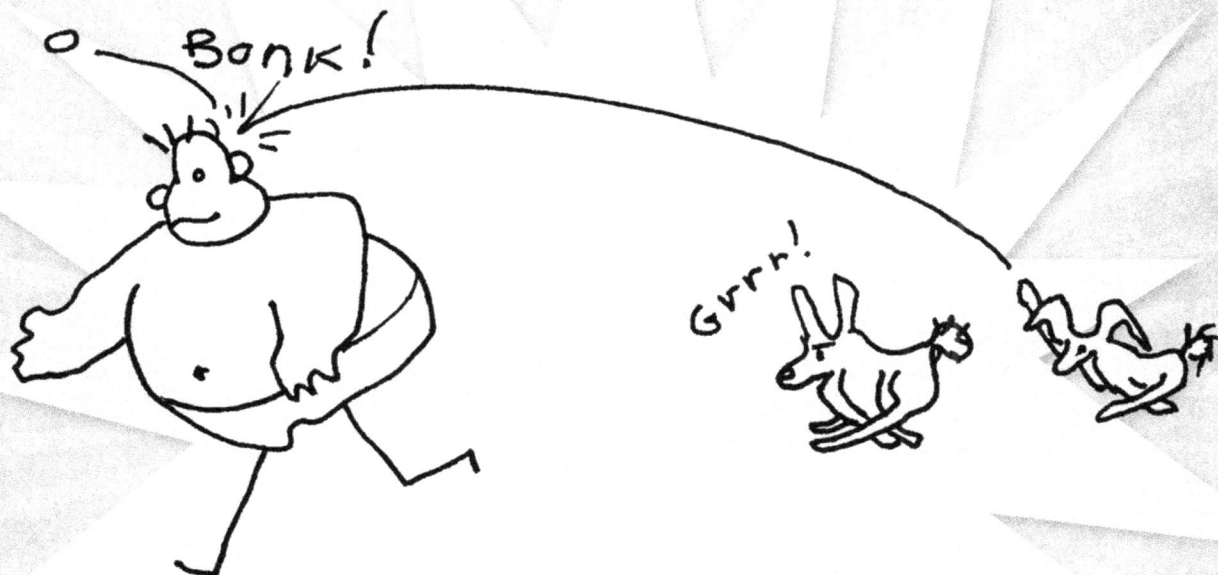

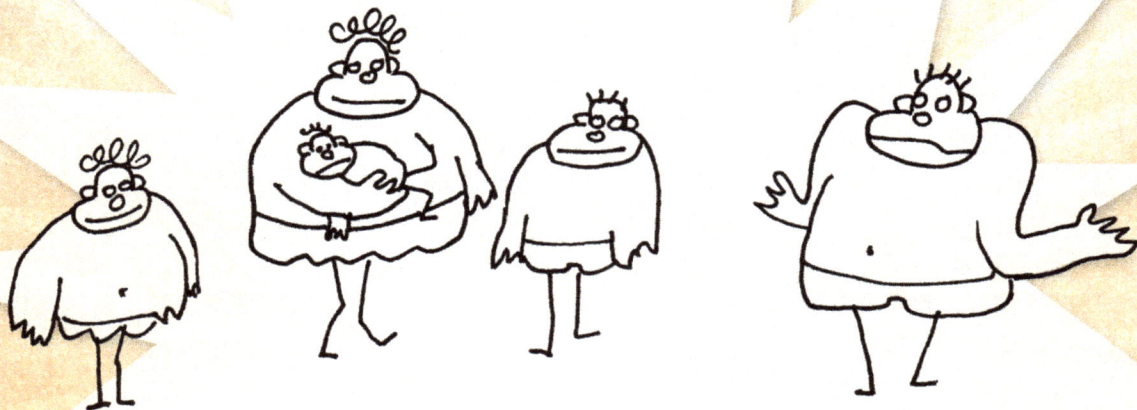

often, he returned foodless.

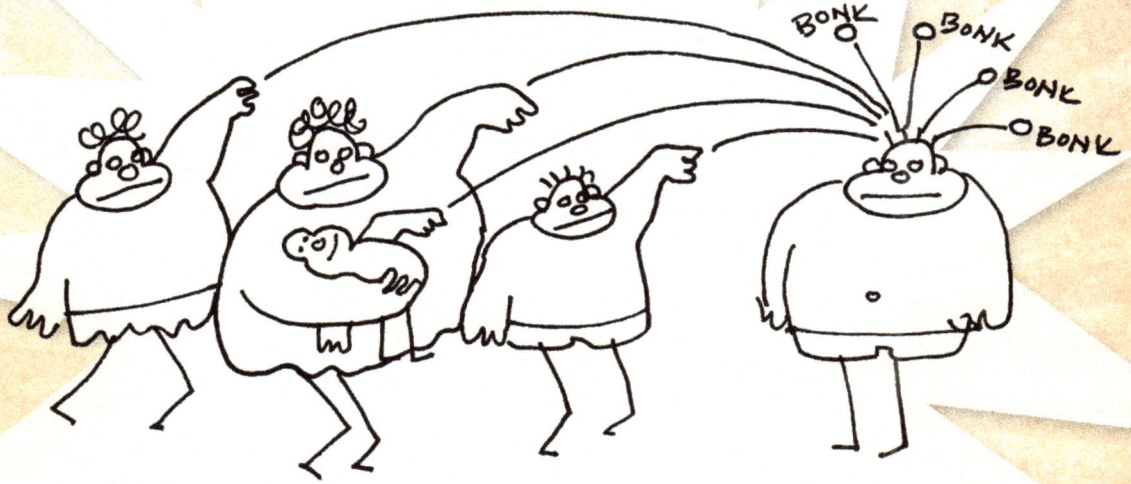

and embarrassed...

9

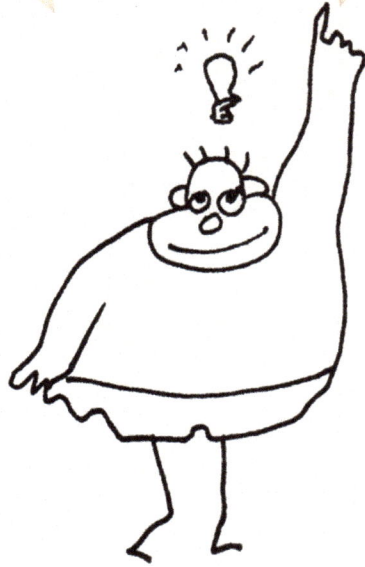

That's when he turned agrarian.

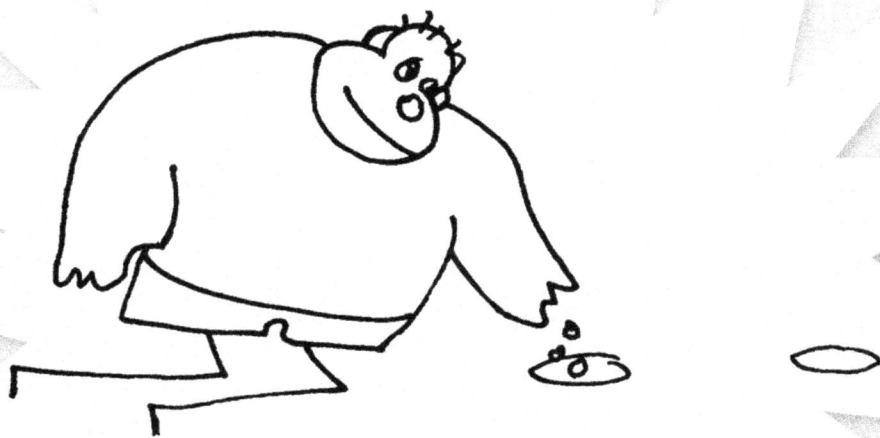

and planted crops.

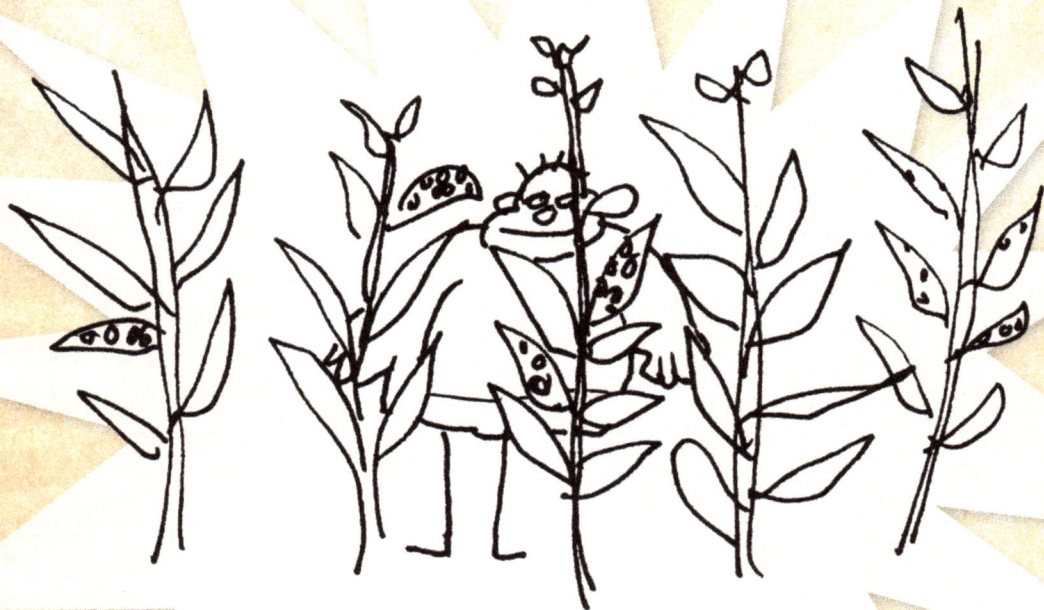

Health food was born.

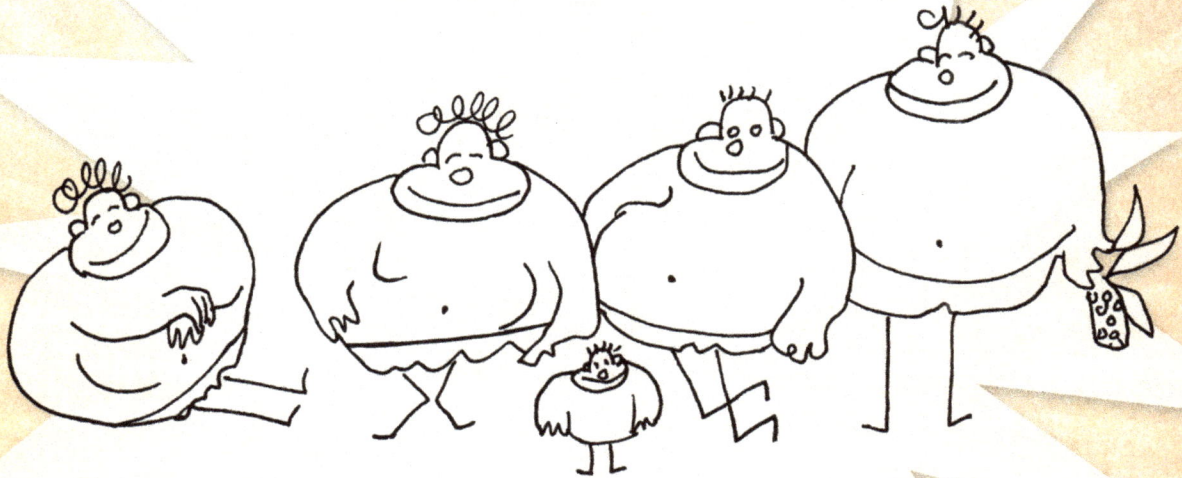

EVERYONE GAINED WEIGHT

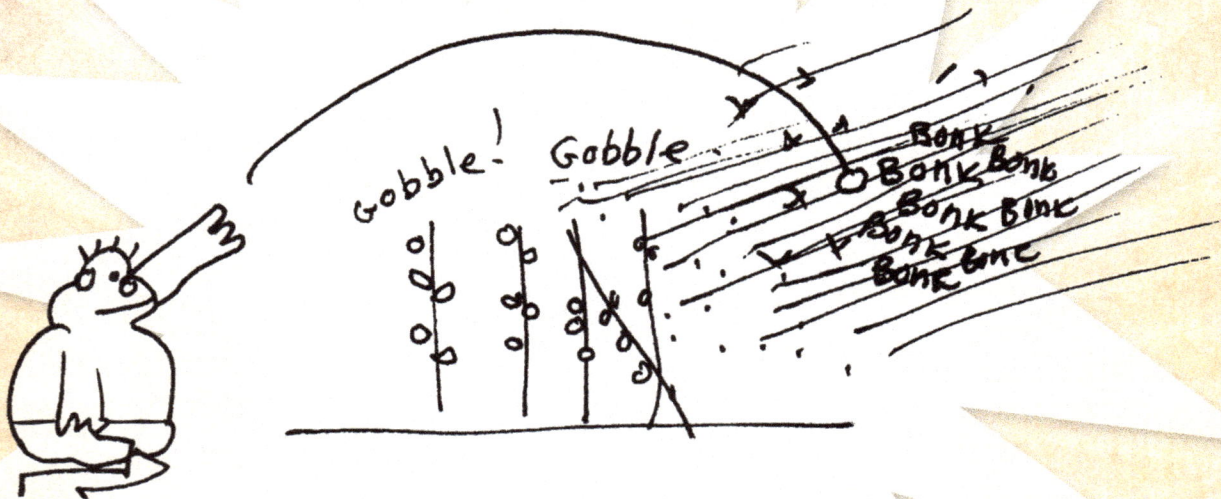

Gobble! Gobble

Bonk
Bonk Bonk
Bonk Bonk
Bonk Bonk
Bonk Bonk

until pestilence. came

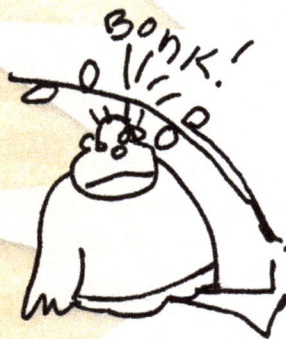

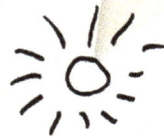

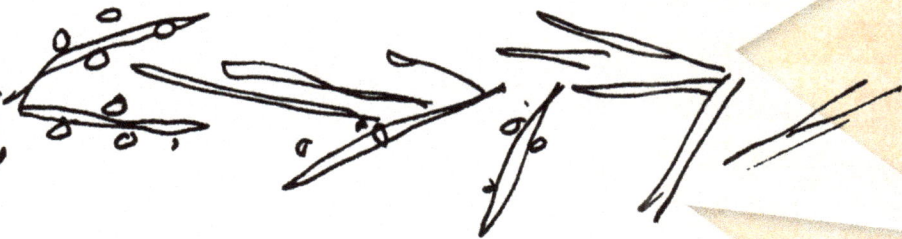

and drought.

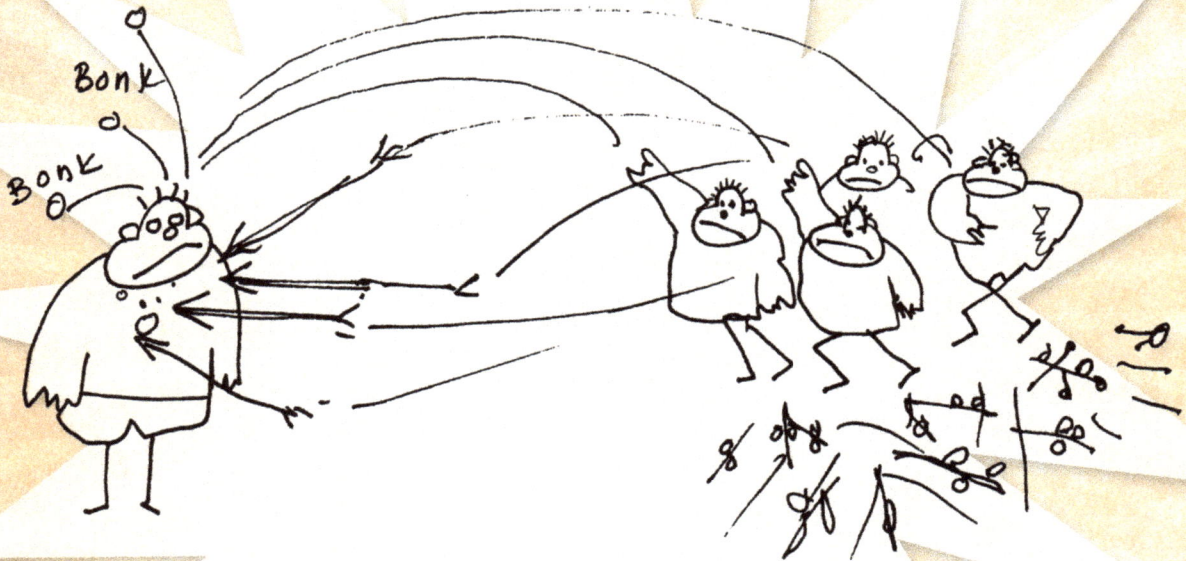

and tribal war.

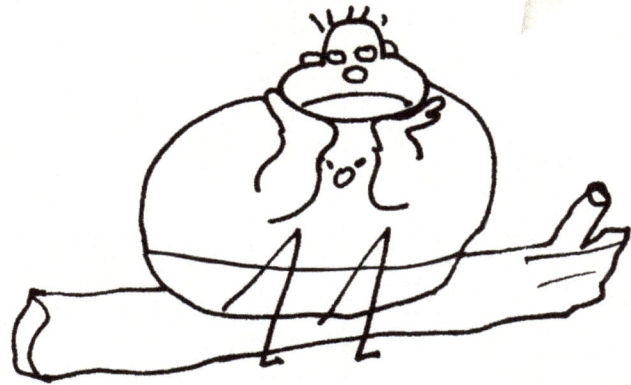

things were not going well.

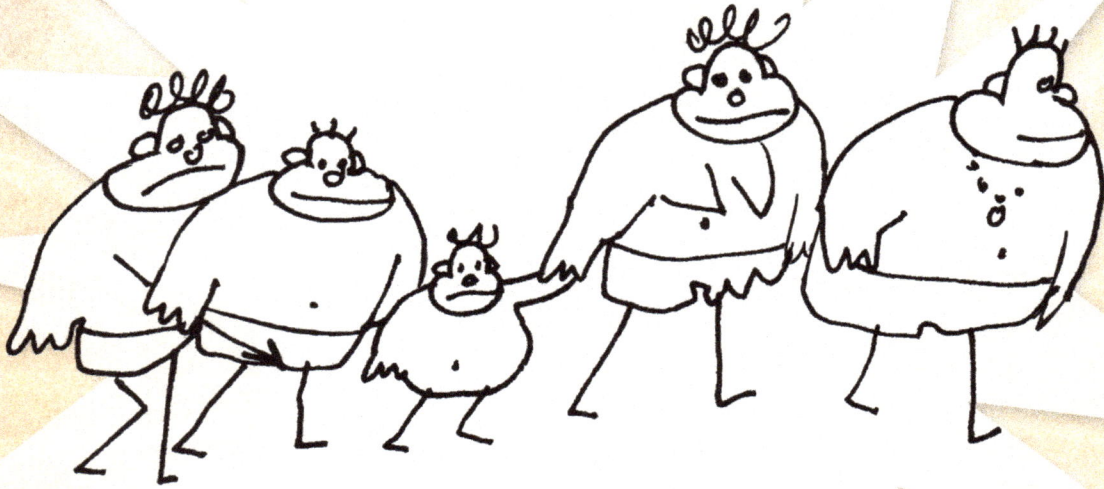

man decided to migrate.

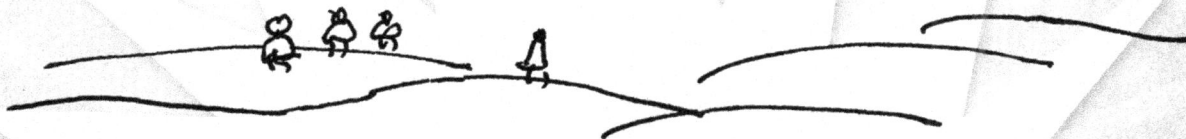

OVER the frozen tundra.

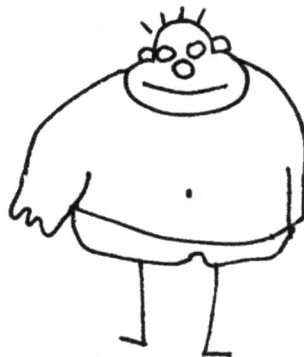

He arrived in America.

19

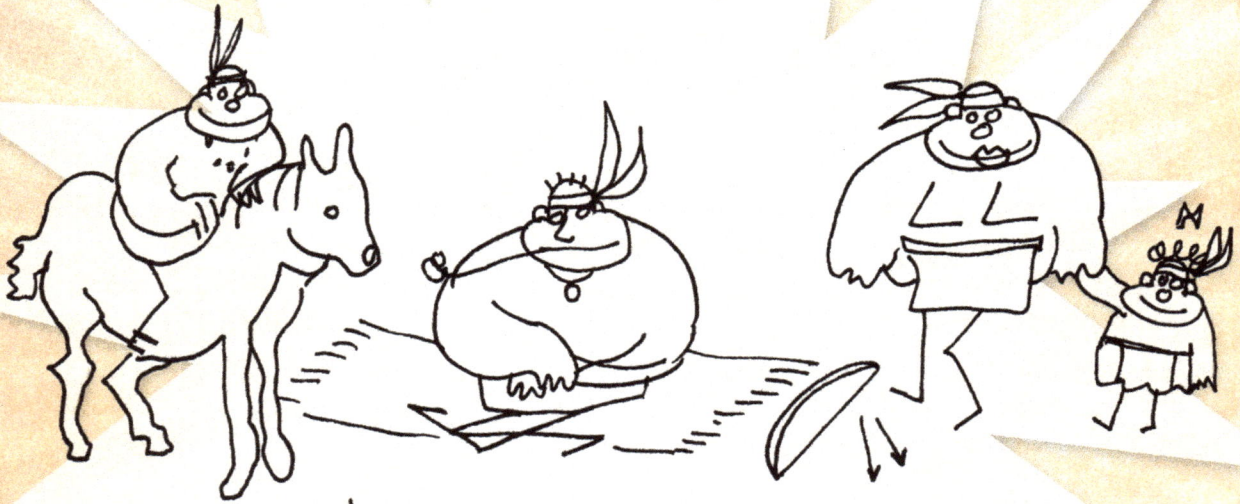

and became indians.

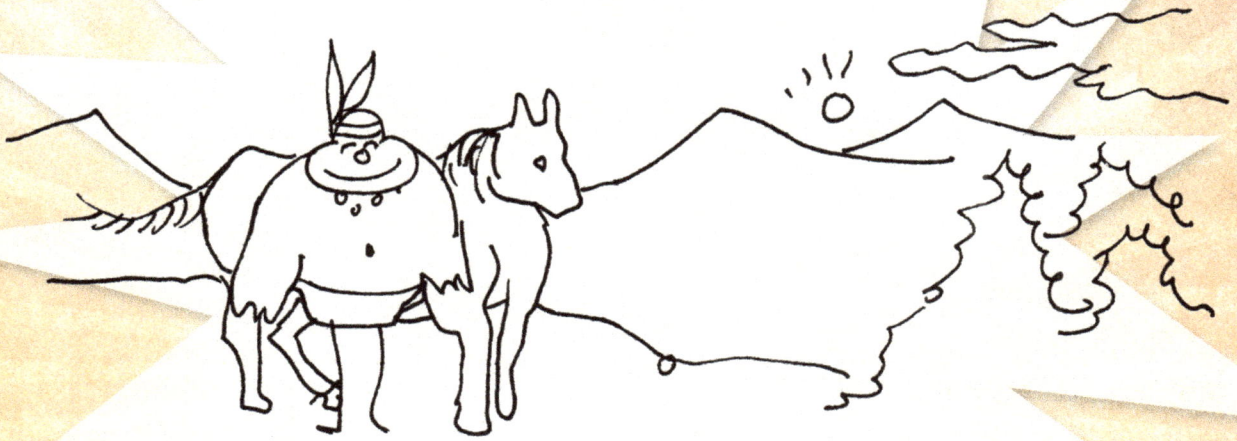

where he lived in peace.

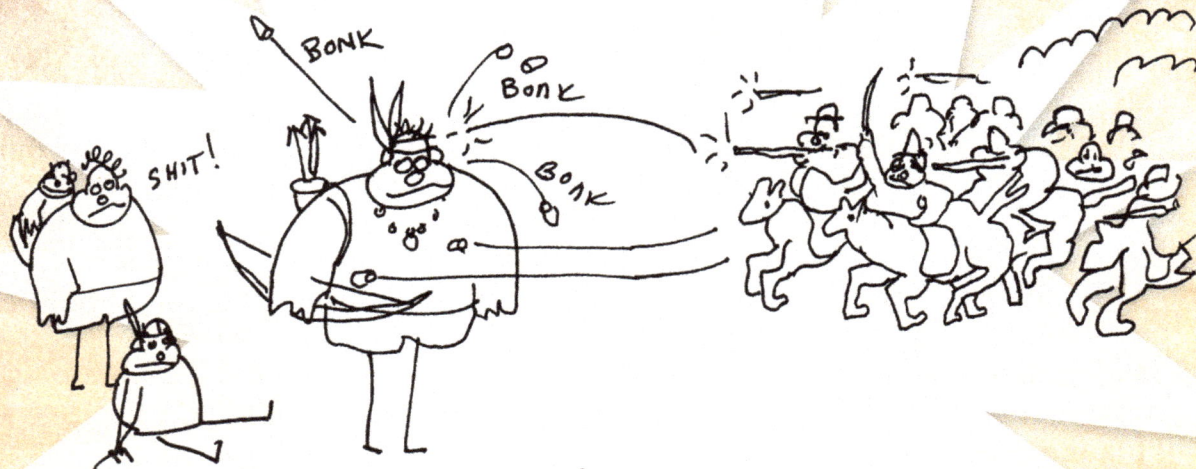

Thoughts for the INTELLIGENT

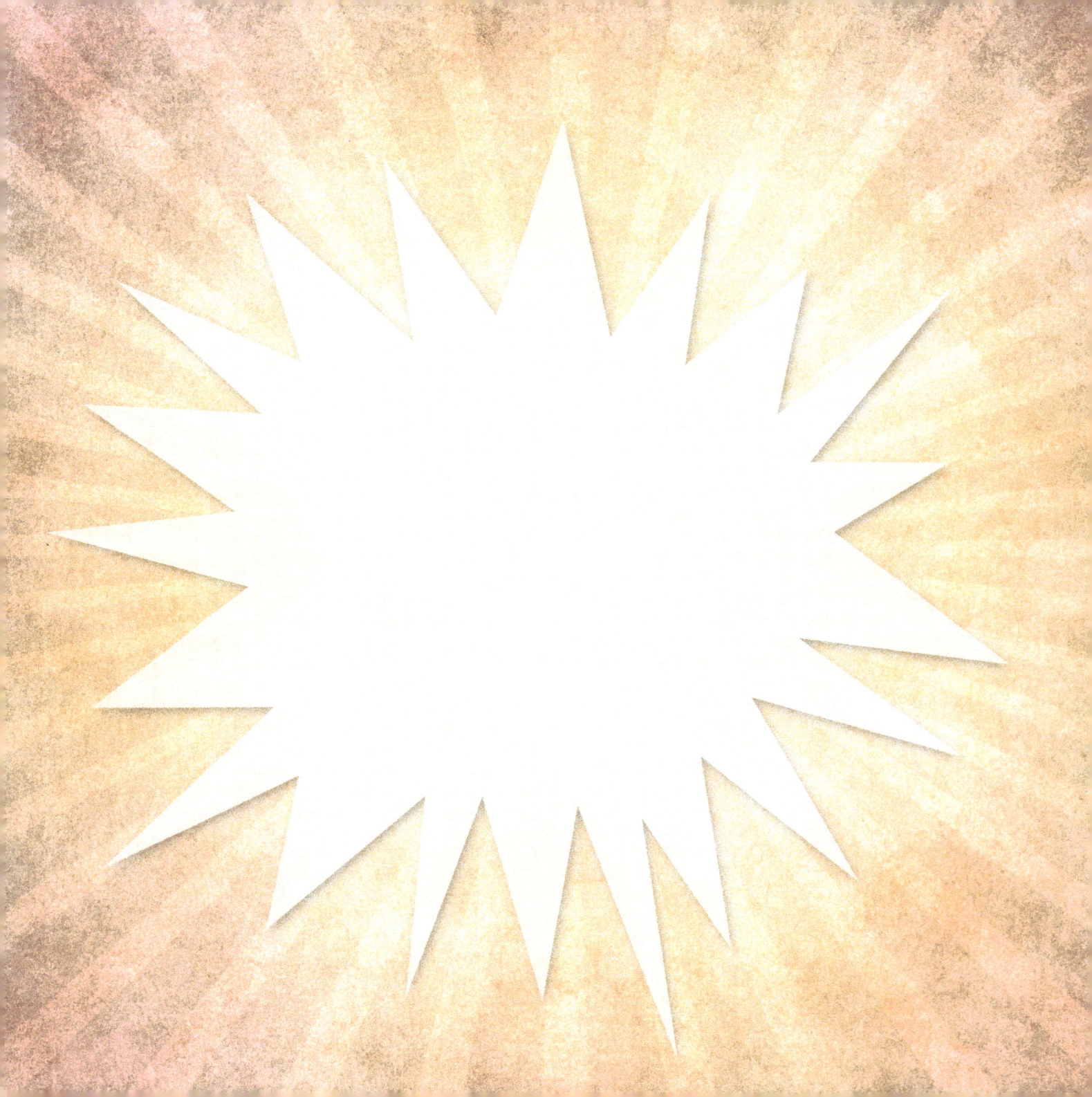

FEEL HOT AND STUFFY?
CAN'T BREATH, CAN'T SEE?
FEEL TRAPPED, UNABLE
TO MOVE ARMS OR CHEST?
FEET ALWAYS ICY COLD?
PERHAPS YOU'RE IN BED BACKWARDS

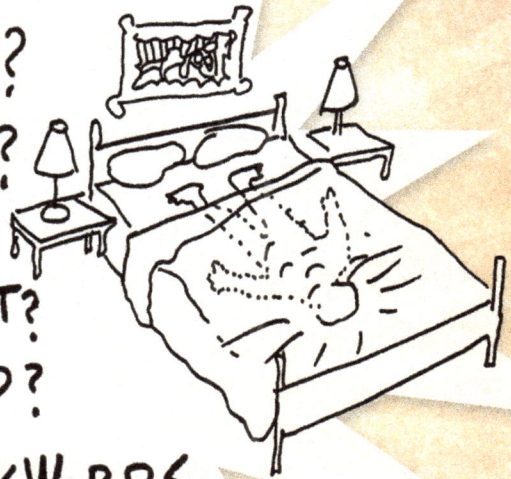

ANSWERS TO OLD QUESTIONS

Q. IF A TREE IN A FOREST FALLS AND MAKES A CRASH AND THERE WAS NO ONE THERE TO HEAR IT, DID IT MAKE A SOUND?

A. ABSOLUTELY, YES. BECAUSE ROY CRANDAL WAS THERE AND HE SAW IT FALL AND HE SAYS "HONEST TO GOD, I HAD MY HANDS OVER MY EARS REAL TIGHT AND I COULD'NT HEAR NOTHING" HOWEVER, HE CAN SEE SOUND, HE SAYS, AND IT REALLY DID MAKE QUITE A RESOUNDING CRASH AS FAR AS HE COULD SEE. SO THAT OUGHT TO PROVE IT. EITHER THAT OR HE'S A BIG LIAR.

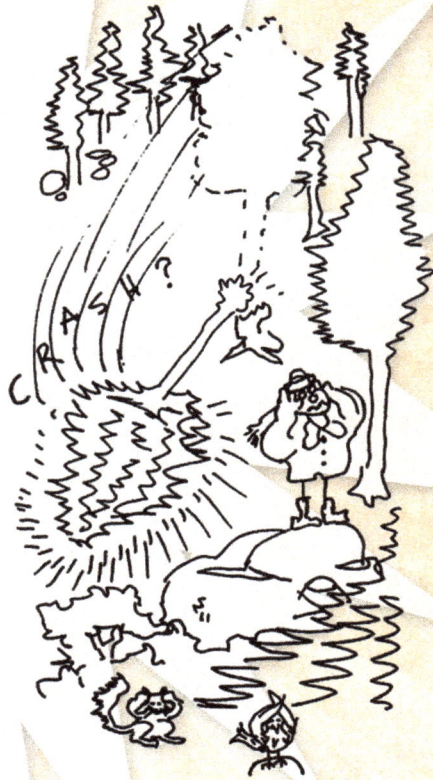

GET YOUR CUSTOMIZED

MANDALA STAMP

CHOOSE FROM $\cancel{5}$ (COUNT 'EM) $\cancel{6}$ 5 DESIGNS.

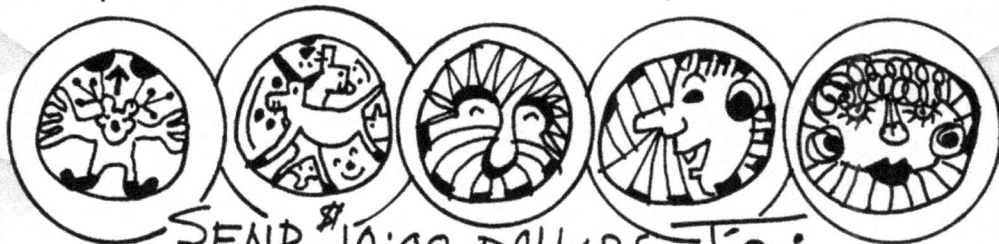

SEND $10:00 DOLLARS TO:

ROY R. CRANDAL

→AT HIS ADDRESS←

TAKE A BLANK SHEET OF PAPER — GET OUT
YOUR MANDALA STAMP - TAKE AIM
WHAM !! YOU GOT A MANDALA
HANG ON WALL OR MEDITATE OR WHATEVER.

ROY R. CRANDAL **FAXOGRAM**

MARKETING IDEA:

SNAP-ON PIE CRUST

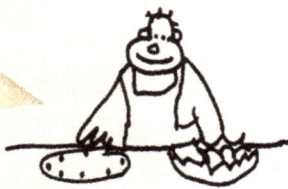 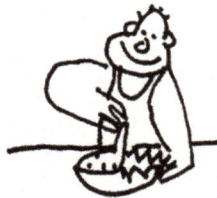 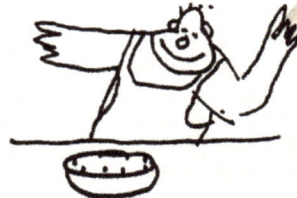

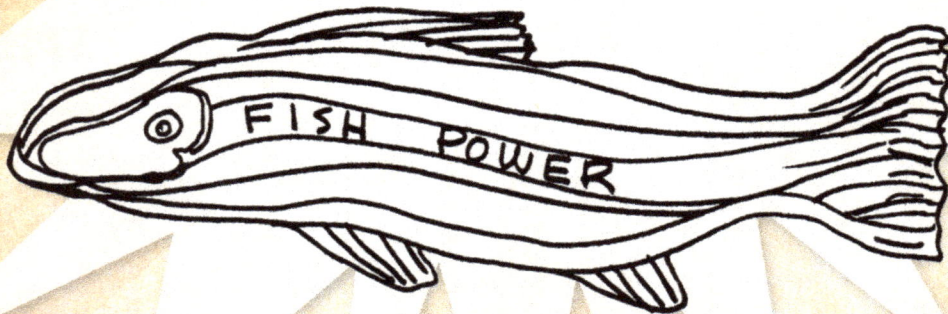

FISH POWER

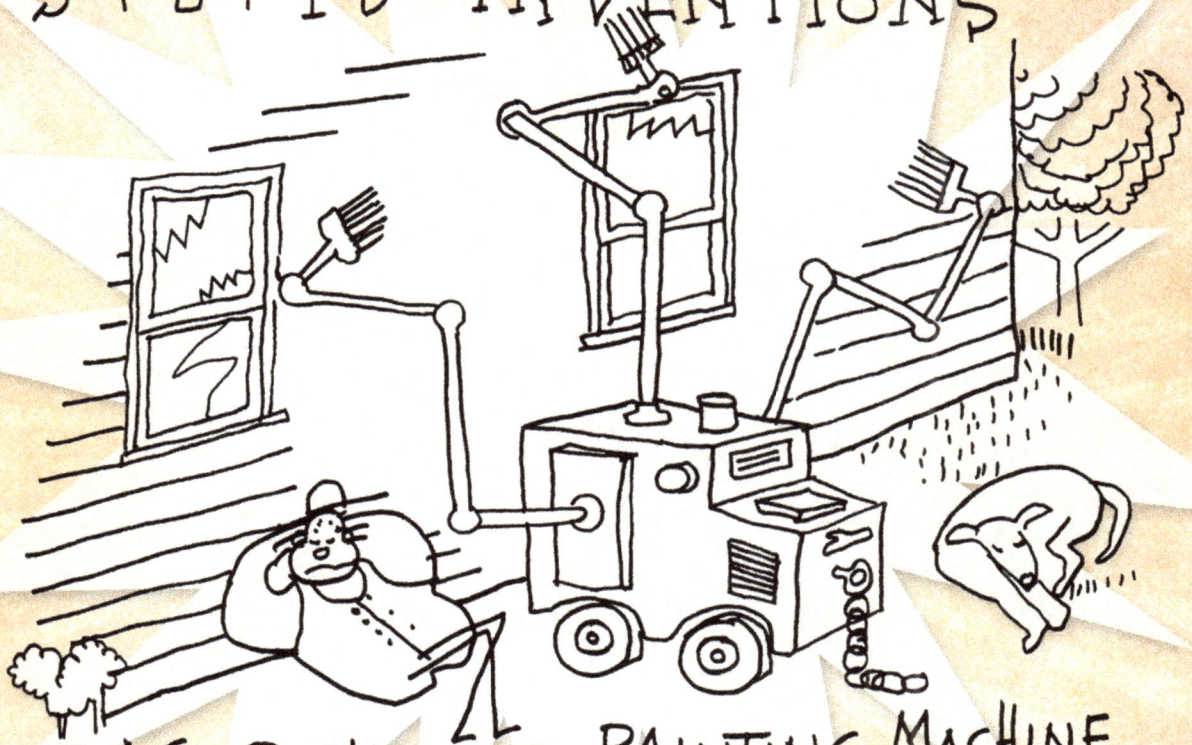

STUPID INVENTIONS

GAS POWERED PAINTING MACHINE

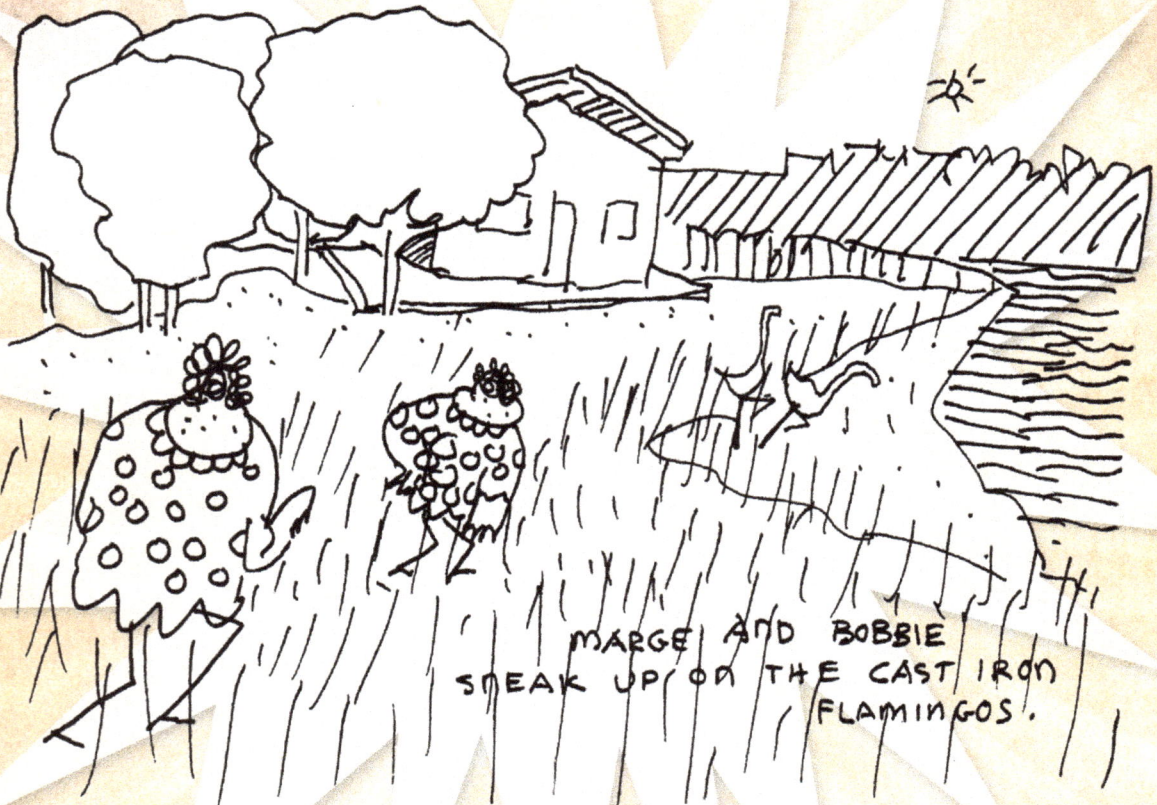

MARGE AND BOBBIE SNEAK UP ON THE CAST IRON FLAMINGOS.

HOW YOU KNOW YOU'RE HERE

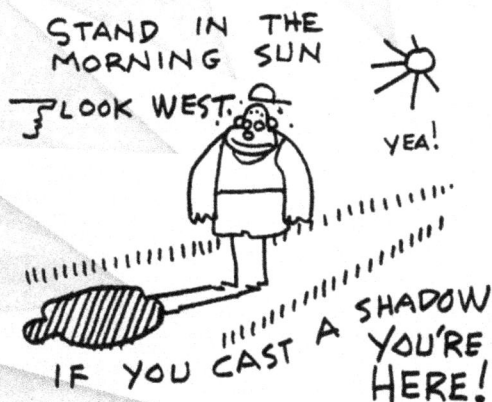

STAND IN THE MORNING SUN. LOOK WEST. YEA!

IF YOU CAST A SHADOW YOU'RE HERE!

GO ALONE TO THE POOL. JUMP IN & OUT REAL FAST. IF THE POOL IS WAVY, YEA! YOU'RE HERE!

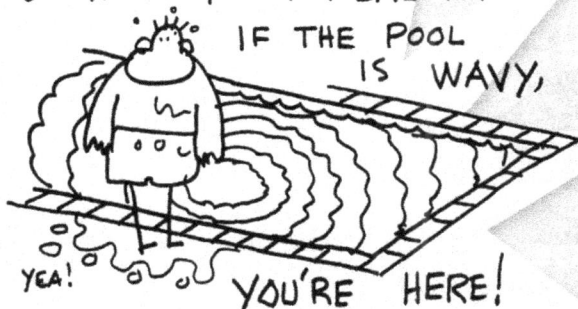

PAY A DOCTOR TO TAKE YOUR PULSE.

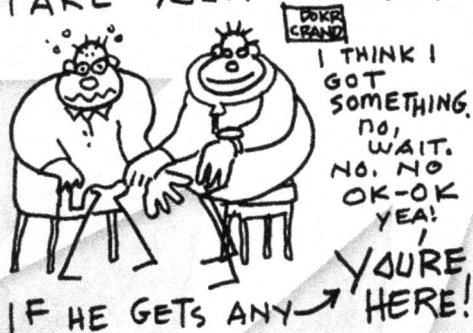

DOKR CRAND

I THINK I GOT SOMETHING. no, WAIT. NO. NO OK-OK YEA!

IF HE GETS ANY → YOU'RE HERE!

TAKE 10 STEPS ON SMOOTH BEACH SAND.

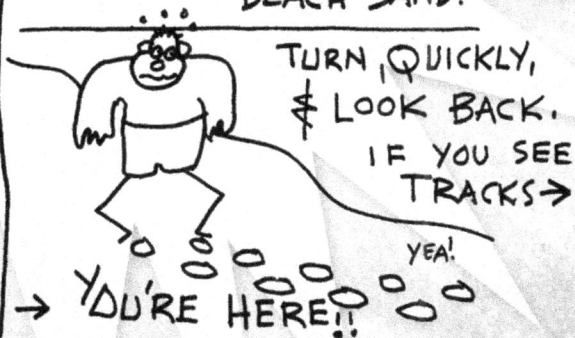

TURN QUICKLY, & LOOK BACK. IF YOU SEE TRACKS → YEA!

→ YOU'RE HERE!!

31

CRANDAL'S
A-Q-PRESSURE
FACELIFT
WITHOUT
SURGERY

LEARN THE KEY
PRESSURE POINTS
ELIMINATE
UNSIGHTLY
FACE LINES

KEY
PRESSURE
POINT
SOME-
WHERE
AROUND
HERE

THE HEART BREAK
OF
UN-
SIGHTLY
FACE
LINES

(POSSIBLY DUE
TO AGE)

☐ Press Special Nerve on face. ☐
I'LL TELL YOU WHERE
IT IS. FOR $10.00.

BE FORE

SEND $10.00
TO ROY CRANDAL
(AT HIS ADDRESS)
AND HE WILL TELL
YOU WHERE THE
SPECIAL NERVE
IS TO PRESS
SO YOU'LL
LOOK LIKE
A NORMAL
PERSON.

ONLY
$10
BIG ONES

THIS IS WHAT
YOU'LL LOOK LIKE
AFTER A-Q-
PRESSURE OF
THE FACE,
SEE? NO UNSIGHTLY
LINES.

⚹HARDLY ANY SIDE
AFFECTS⚹
FOR ONE
DOLLAR MORE YOU
GET SIDE AFFECT ANTIDOTE.

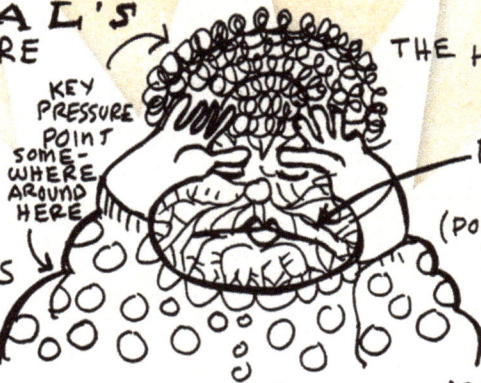

AFTER

LOOK LIKE
THE REST
OF US!
FOR
ONLY 10
BUCKS!
IF YOU DON'T TRUST
IT, PRACTICE ON
A PRUNE, FIRST.

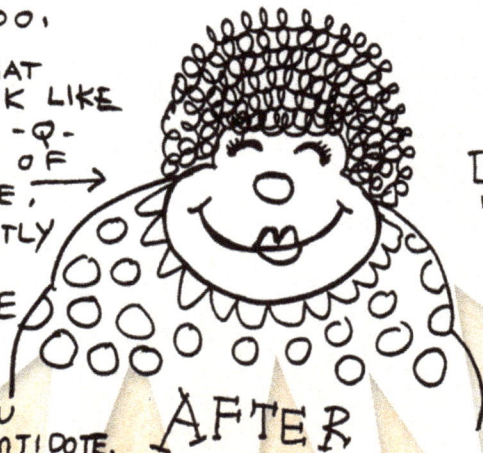

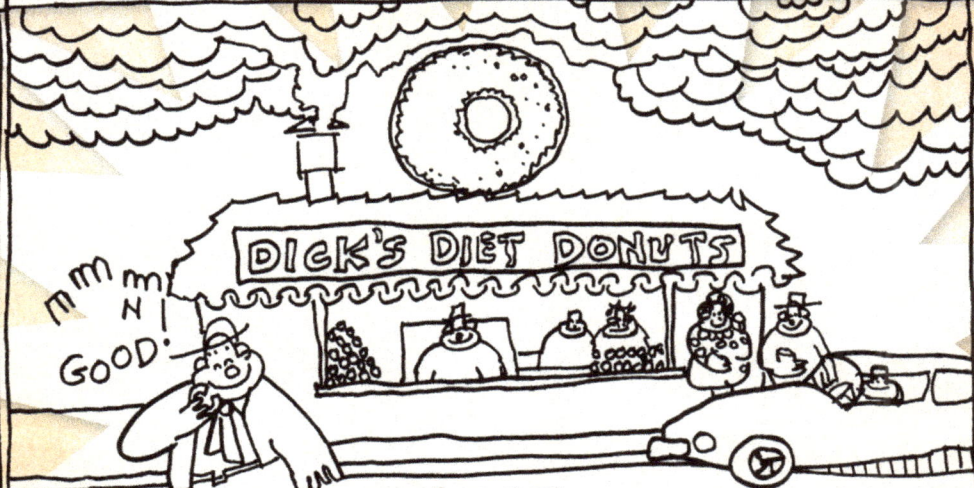

PRE - THINKING

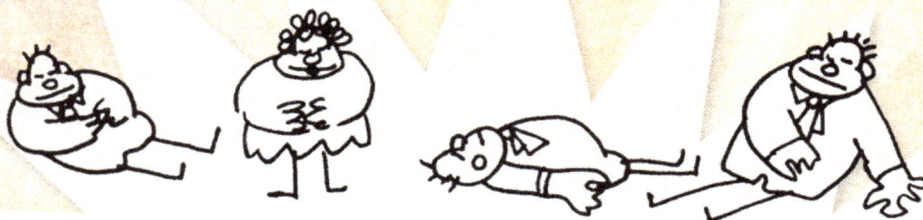

THINKING

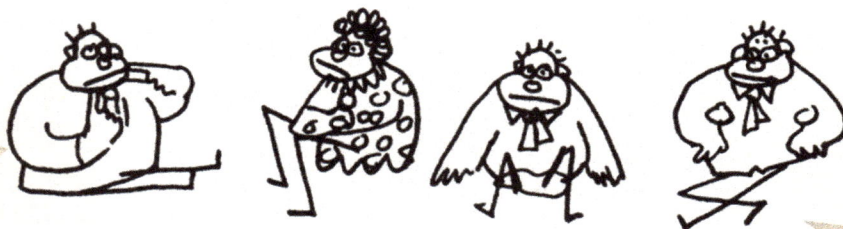

ACTION

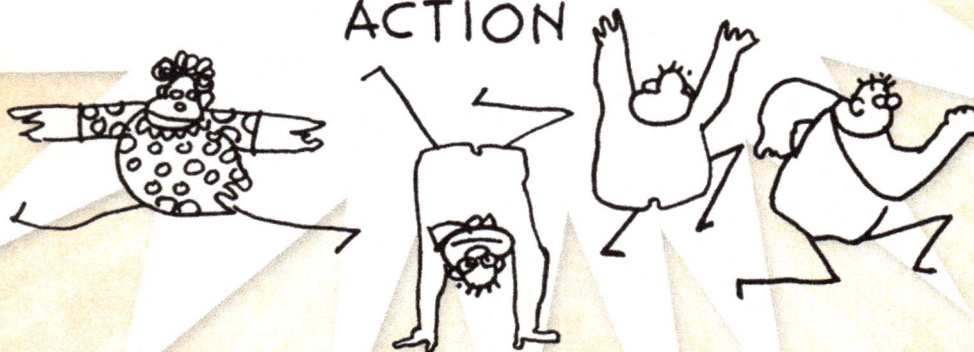

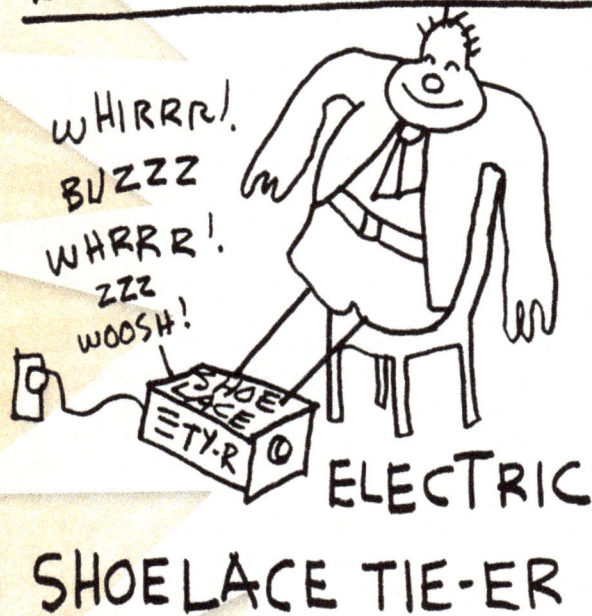
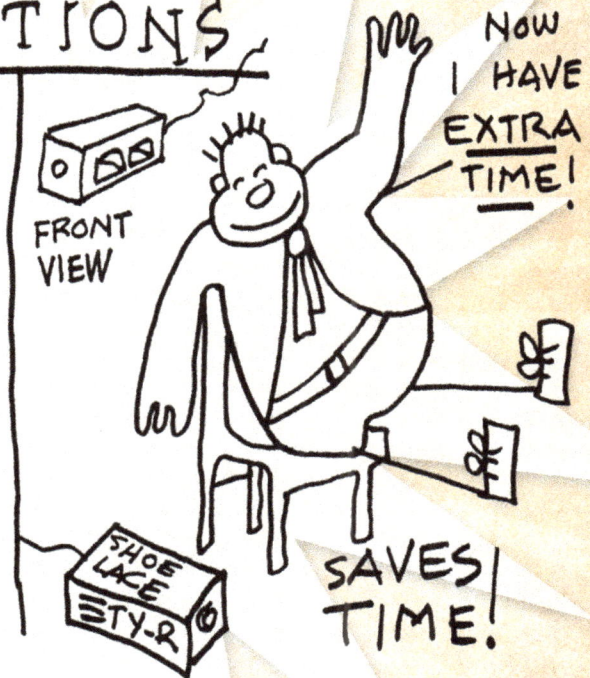

CRANDAL TIPS

DON'T GET COOKIES ON YOUR CD
WHEN EATING COOKIES AND CRUMBS
FALL ON THE "BUSINESS" SIDE OF
YOUR CD JUST BEFORE IT DISAPPEARS
INTO THE LITTLE SLOT, YOU MAY BE
IN TROUBLE. YOU'LL GUM UP THE WORKS!
THE MUSIC WILL SOUND BUMPY AS IT
GETS IN WAY OF THE LIGHT. YOU
WILL ADD LASER LIGHT FRICTION.
YOUR DISC WILL SOUND FUZZY.
YOU MAY HAVE TO GET A NEW
LIGHT. IF YOU'RE PLAYING
YOUR CD AND IT SOUNDS
BUMPY OR FUZZY, CHECK
FOR COOKIES ON THE C.D.

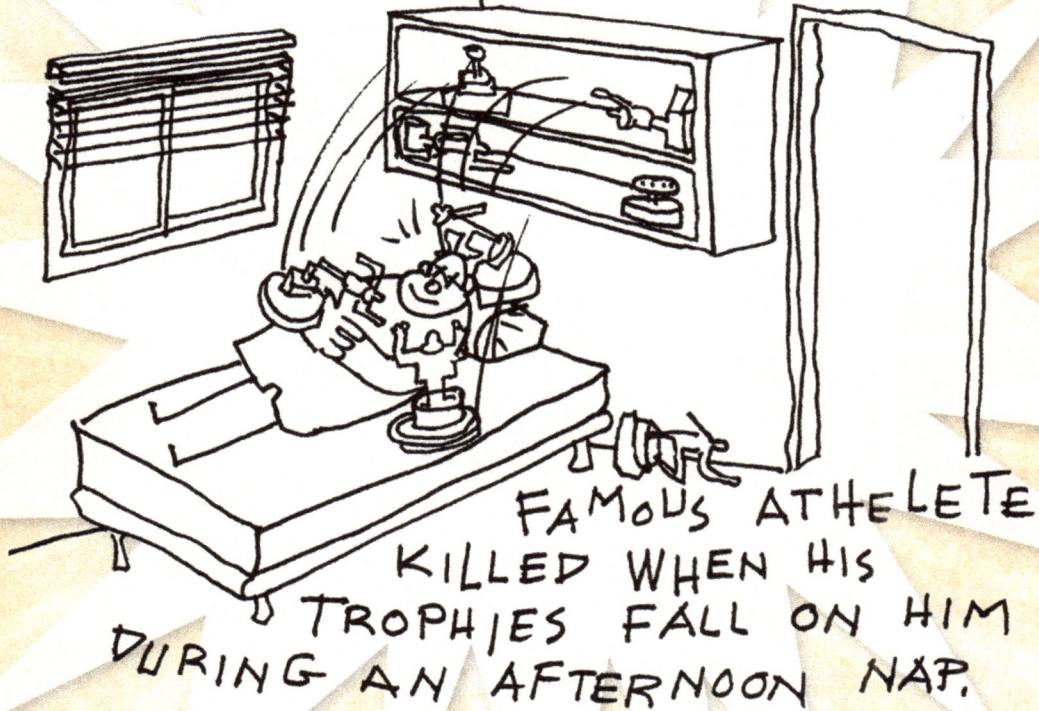

IRONIC DEATHS

FAMOUS ATHELETE KILLED WHEN HIS TROPHIES FALL ON HIM DURING AN AFTERNOON NAP.

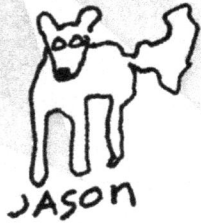

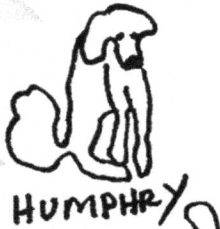

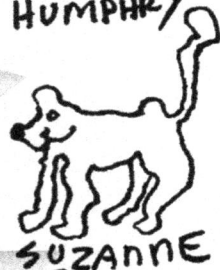

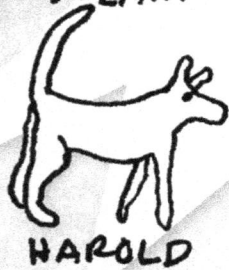

JASON

HUMPHRY

SUZANNE

HAROLD

A-HUH!.

R UH-UN UH-UH
VH-UH

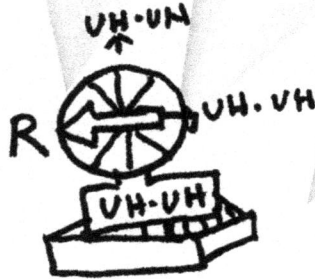

Send 10 dollars to Roy R Crandal AND HE WILL SEND YOU THE

ALL WEATHER KITCHEN
GUARANTEED COMPASS
(ALWAYS POINTS TO THE REFRIGERATOR)

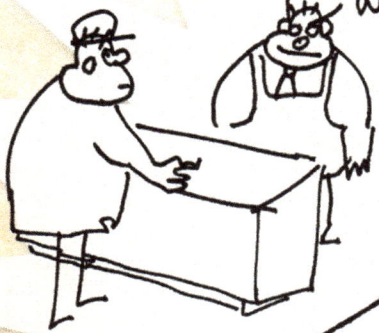

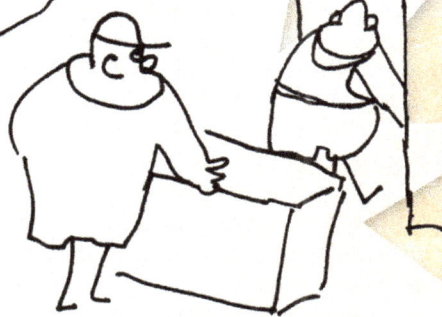

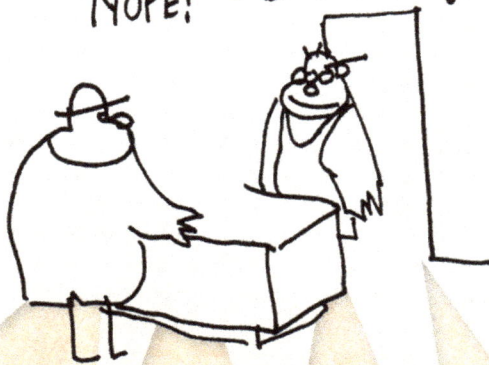

39

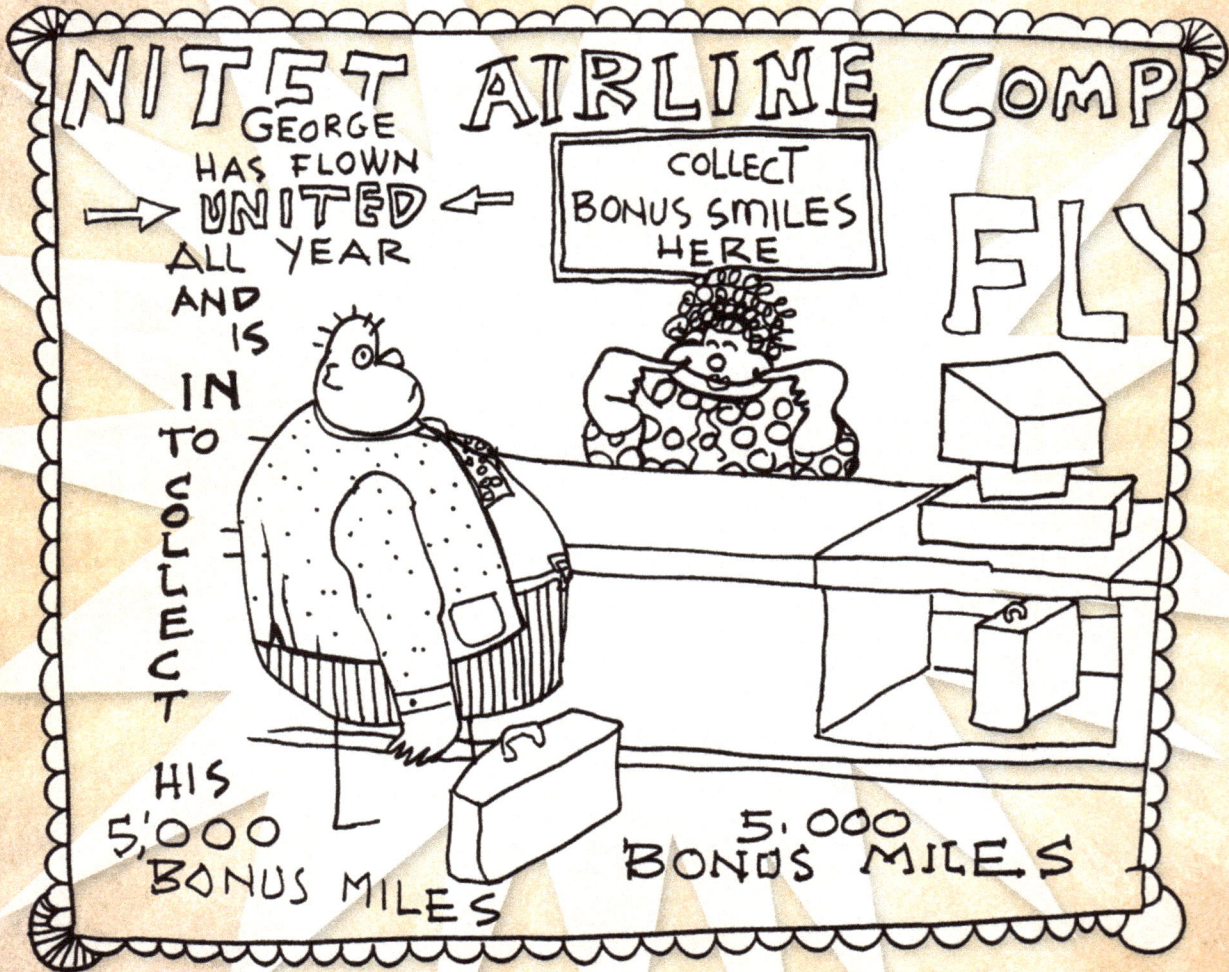

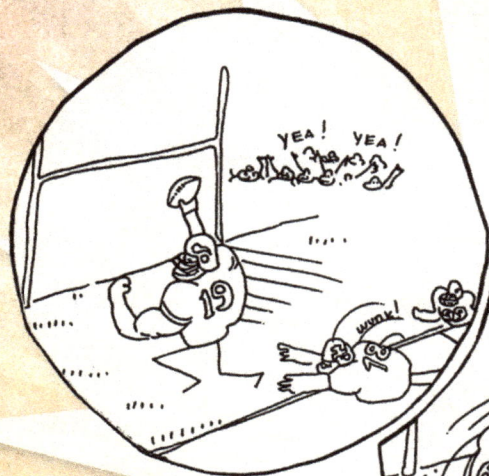
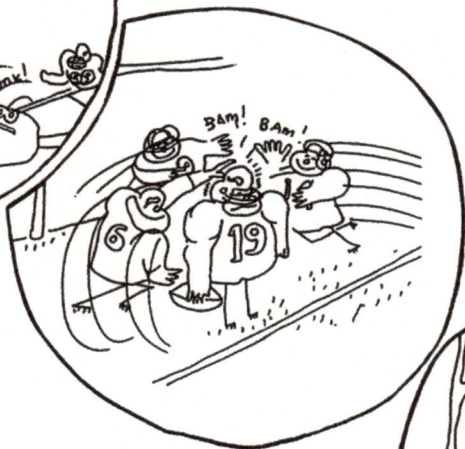
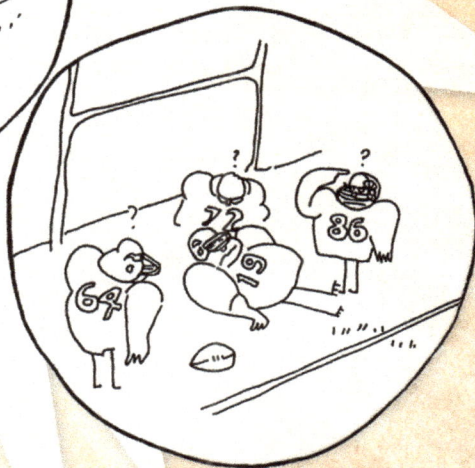

41

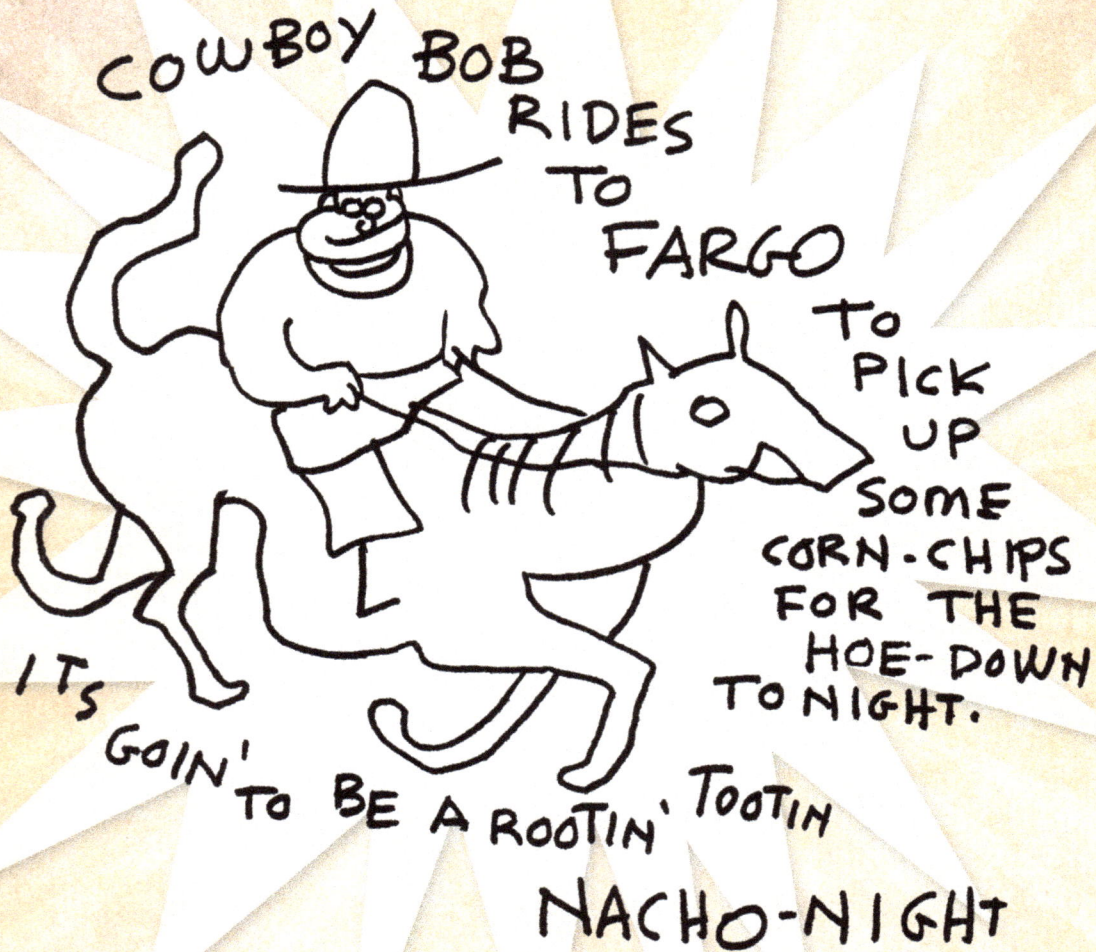

COWBOY BOB RIDES TO FARGO TO PICK UP SOME CORN-CHIPS FOR THE HOE-DOWN TONIGHT.

IT'S GOIN' TO BE A ROOTIN' TOOTIN' NACHO-NIGHT

42

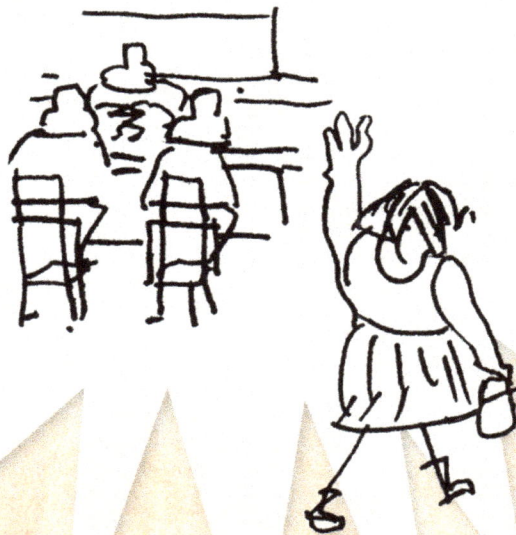

THE DANCE
OR
WHA' HOPPEN!

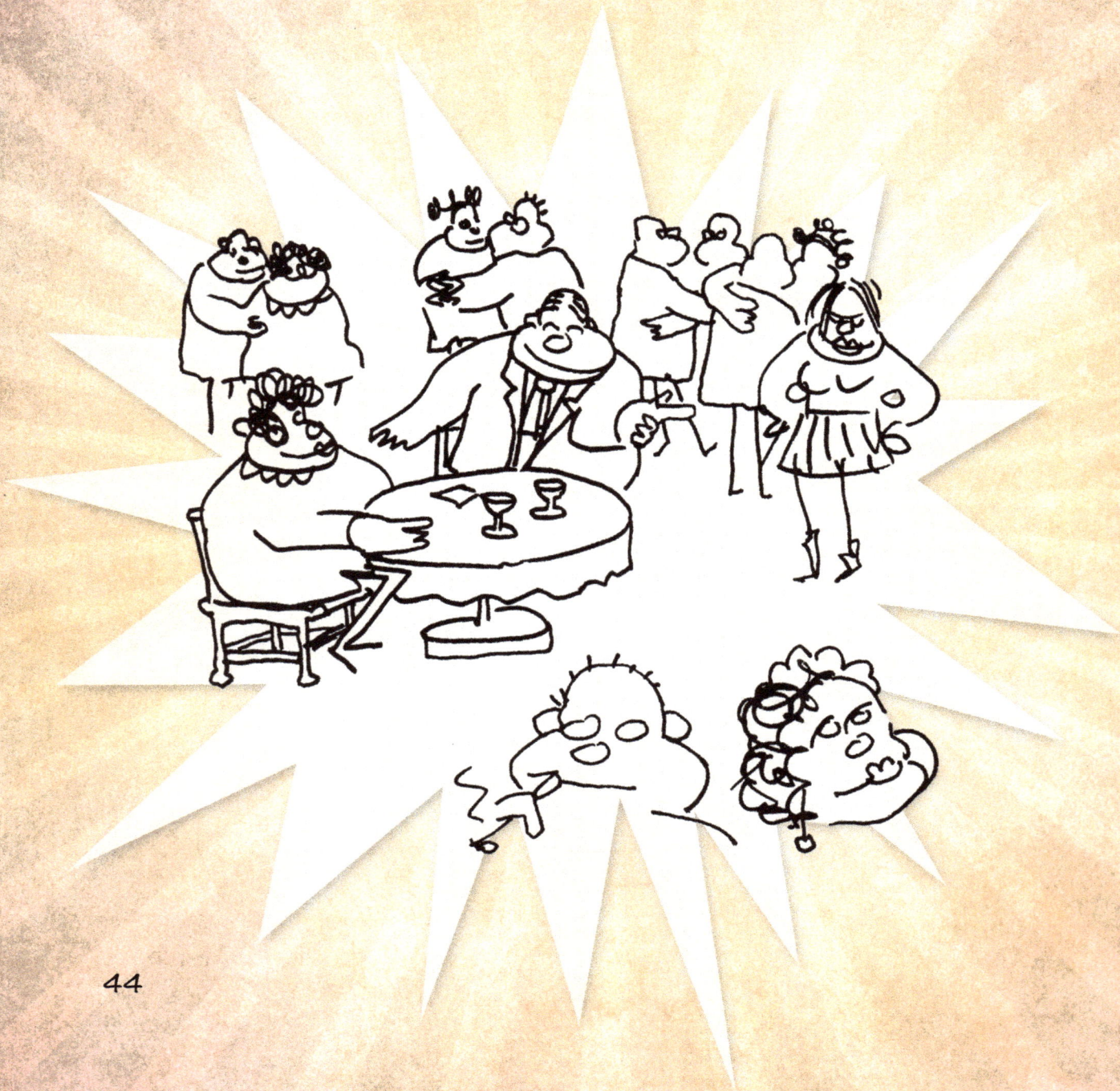

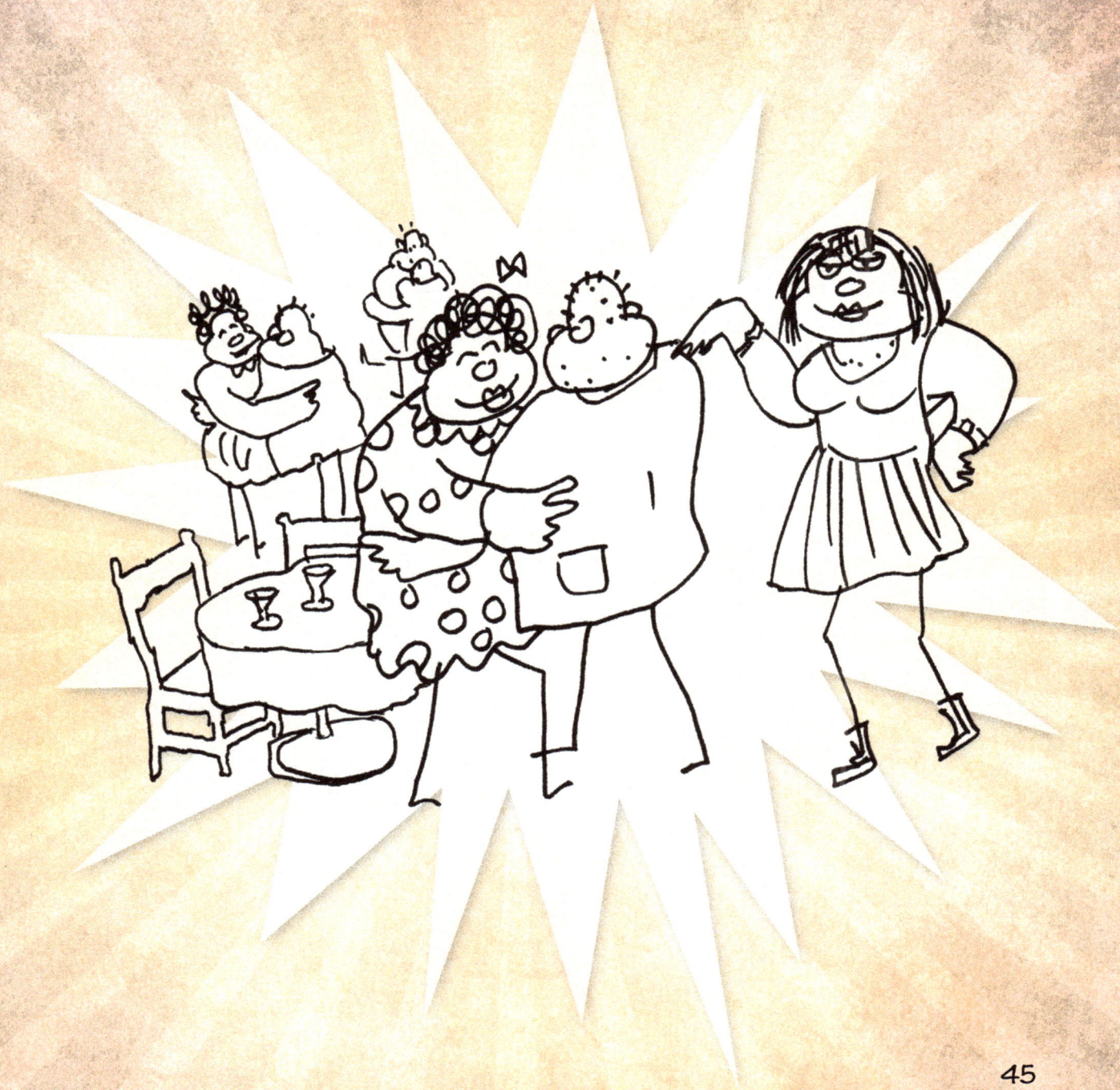

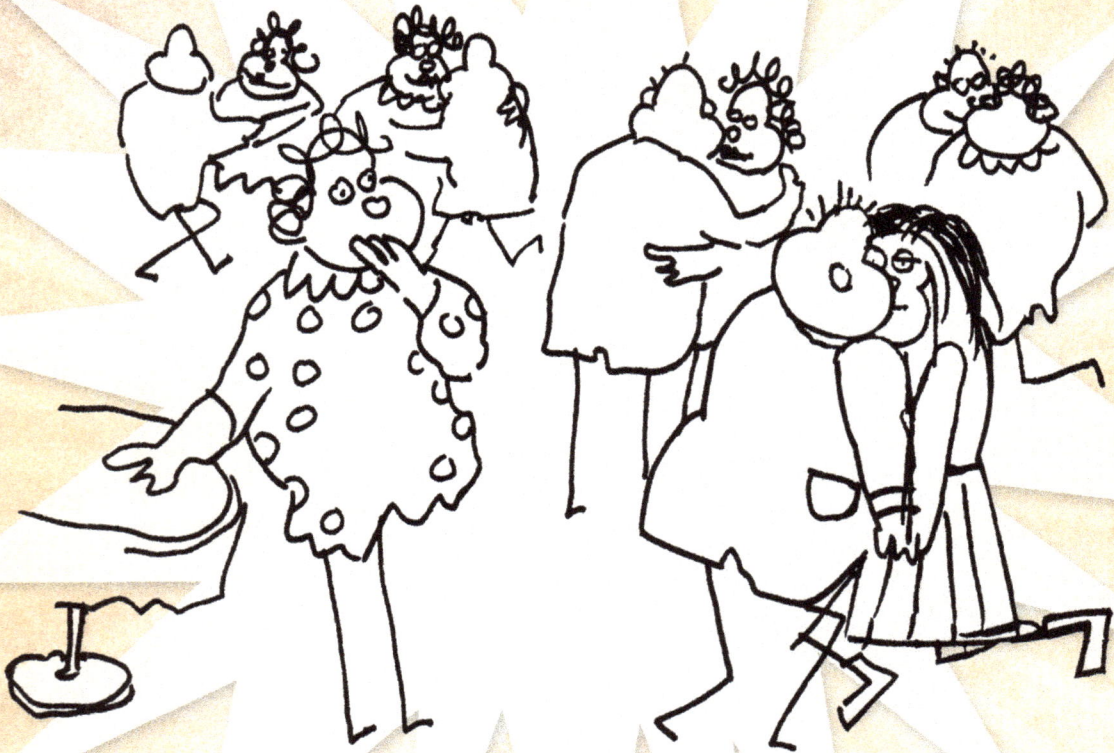

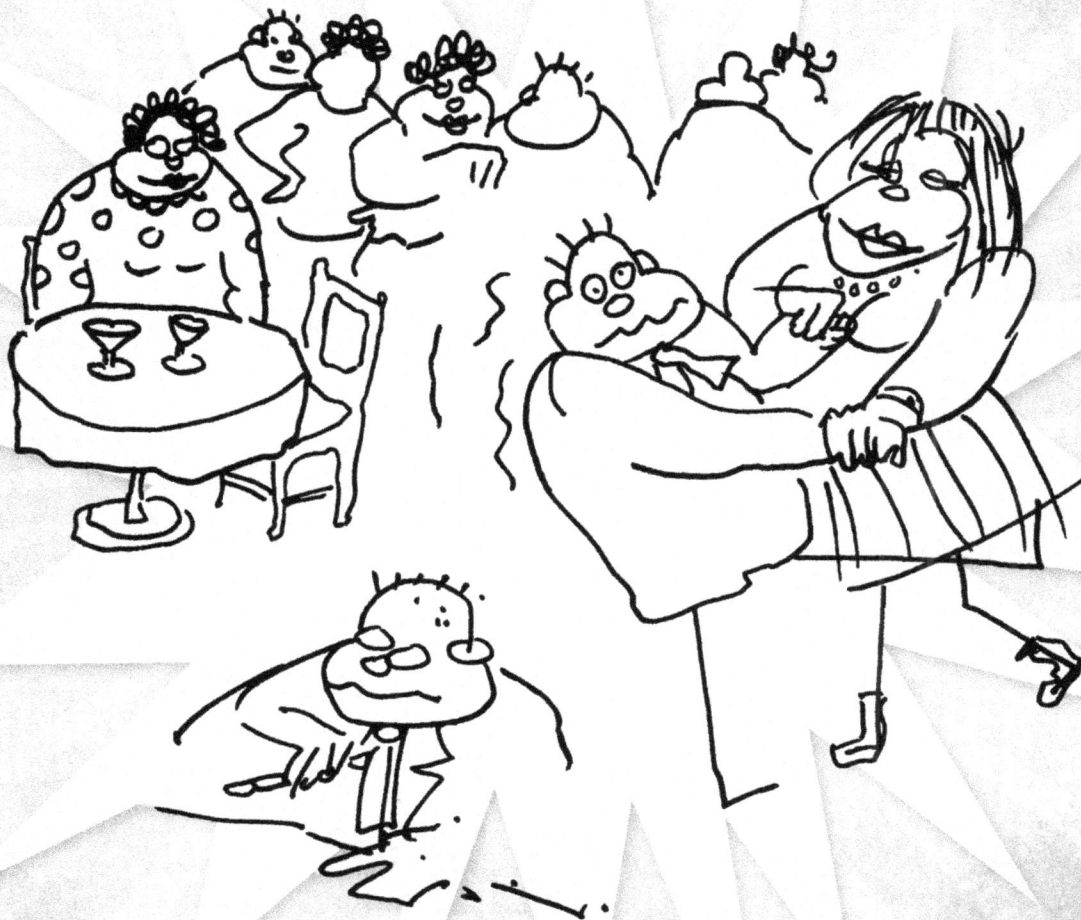

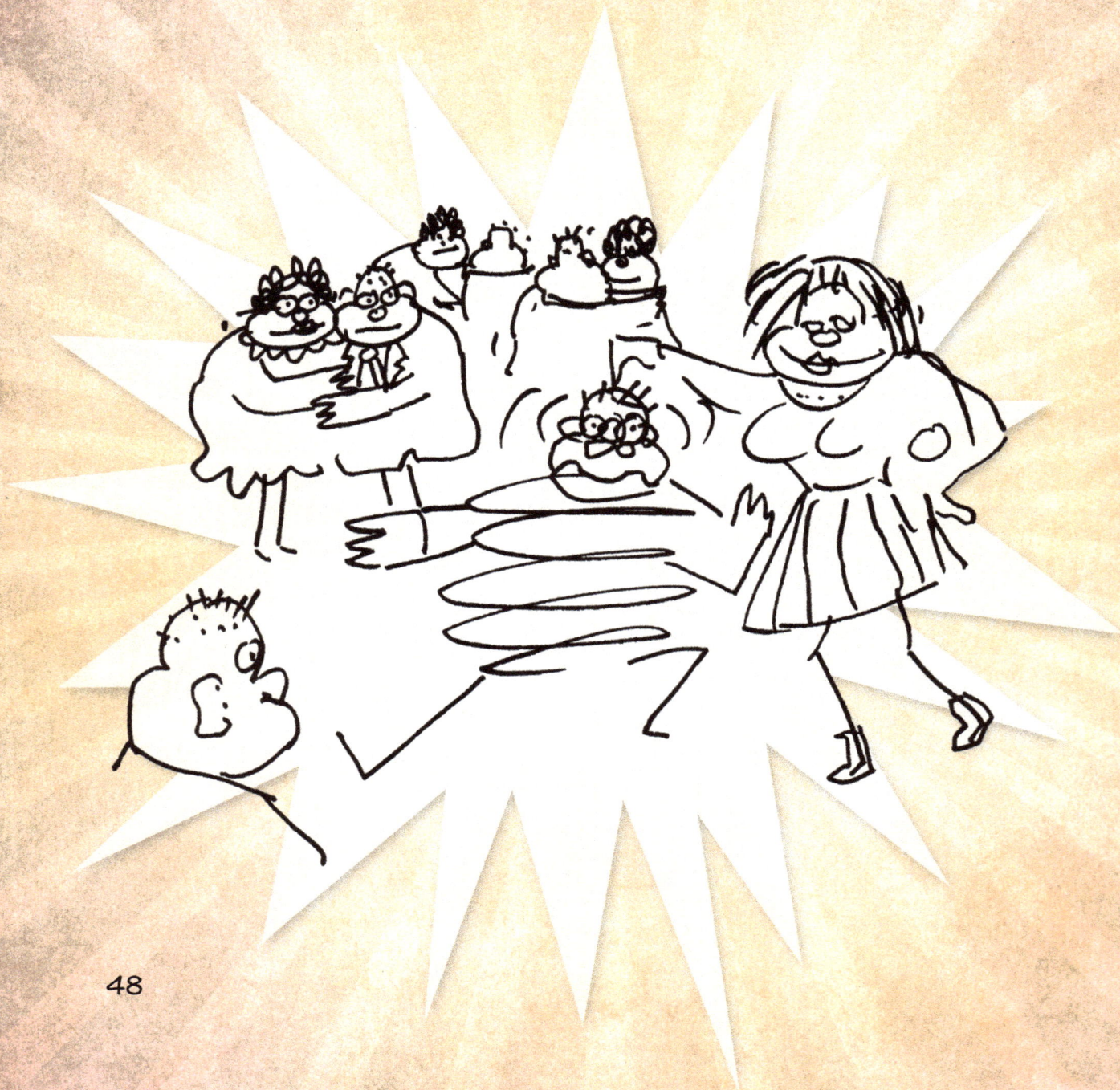

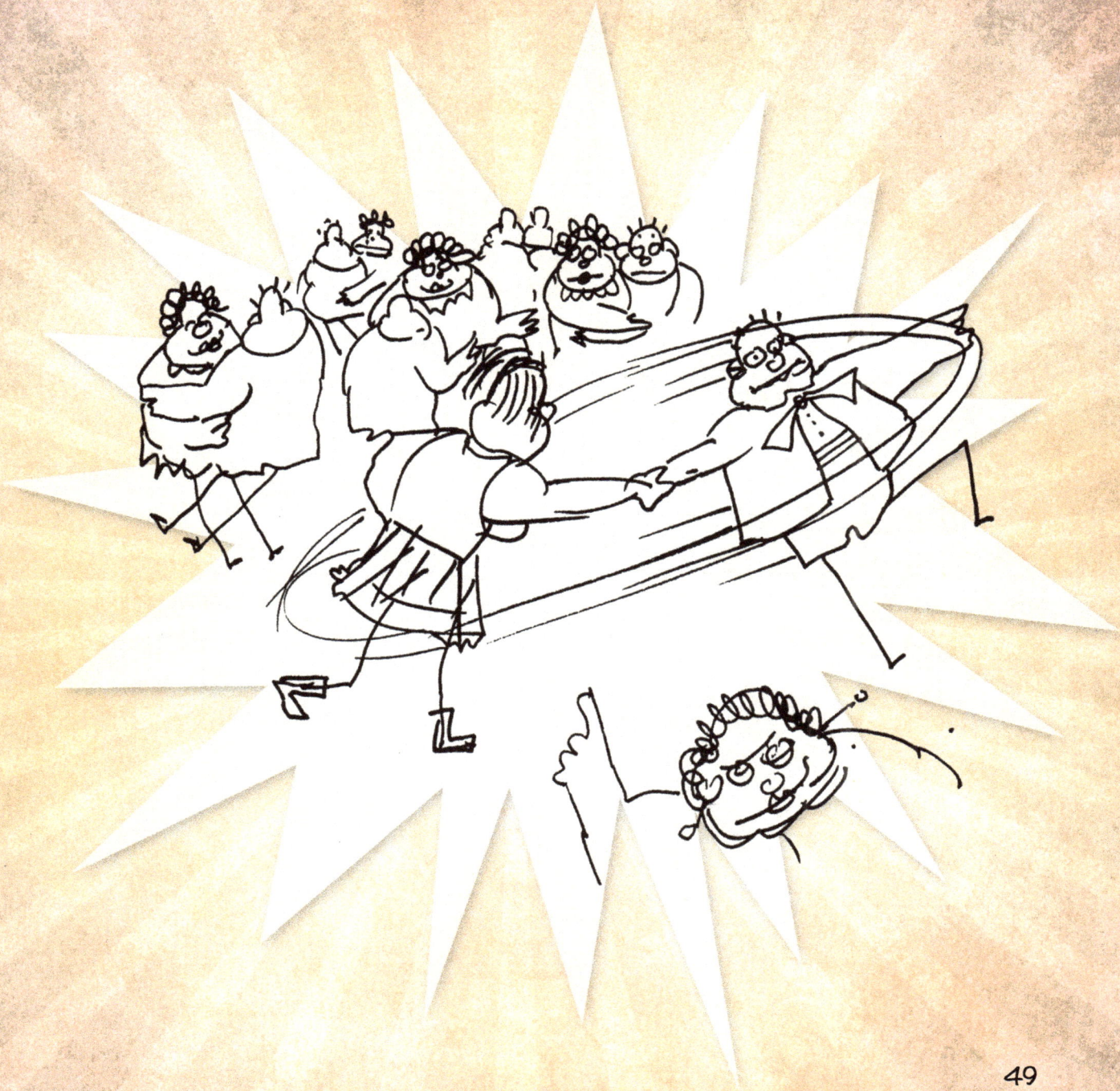

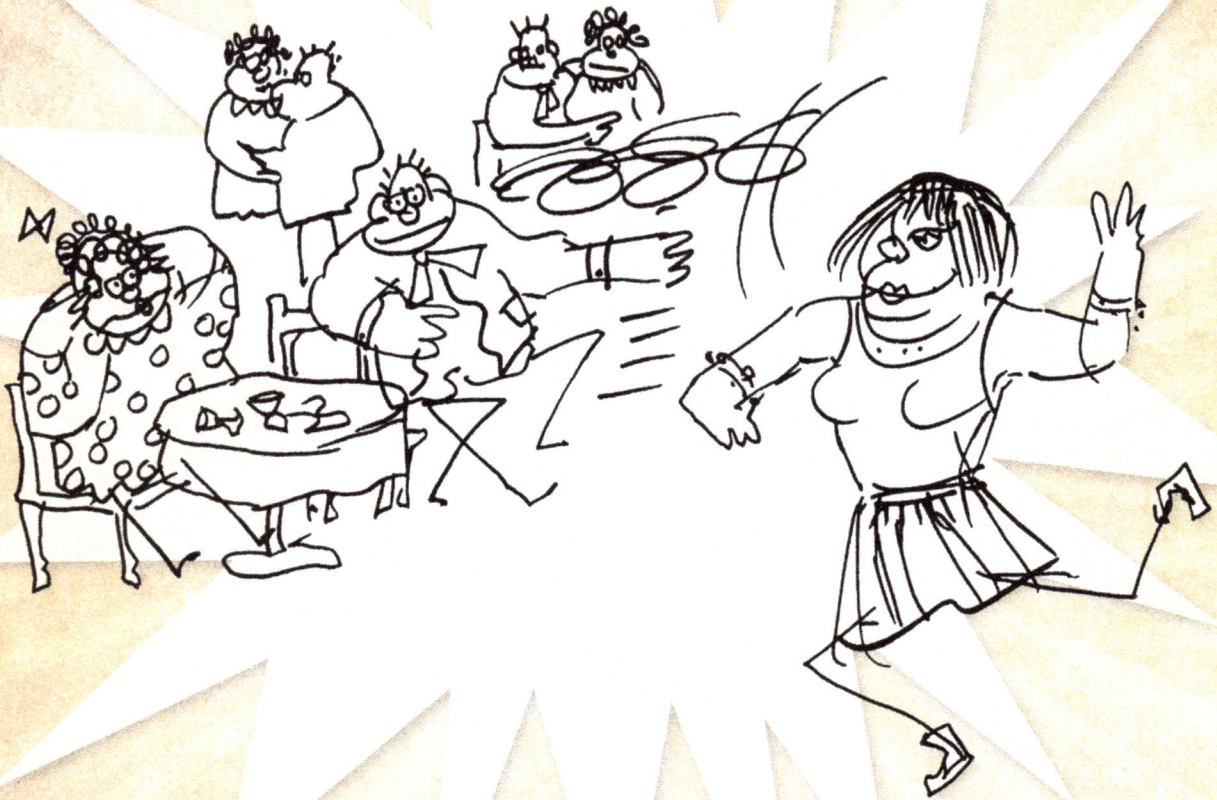

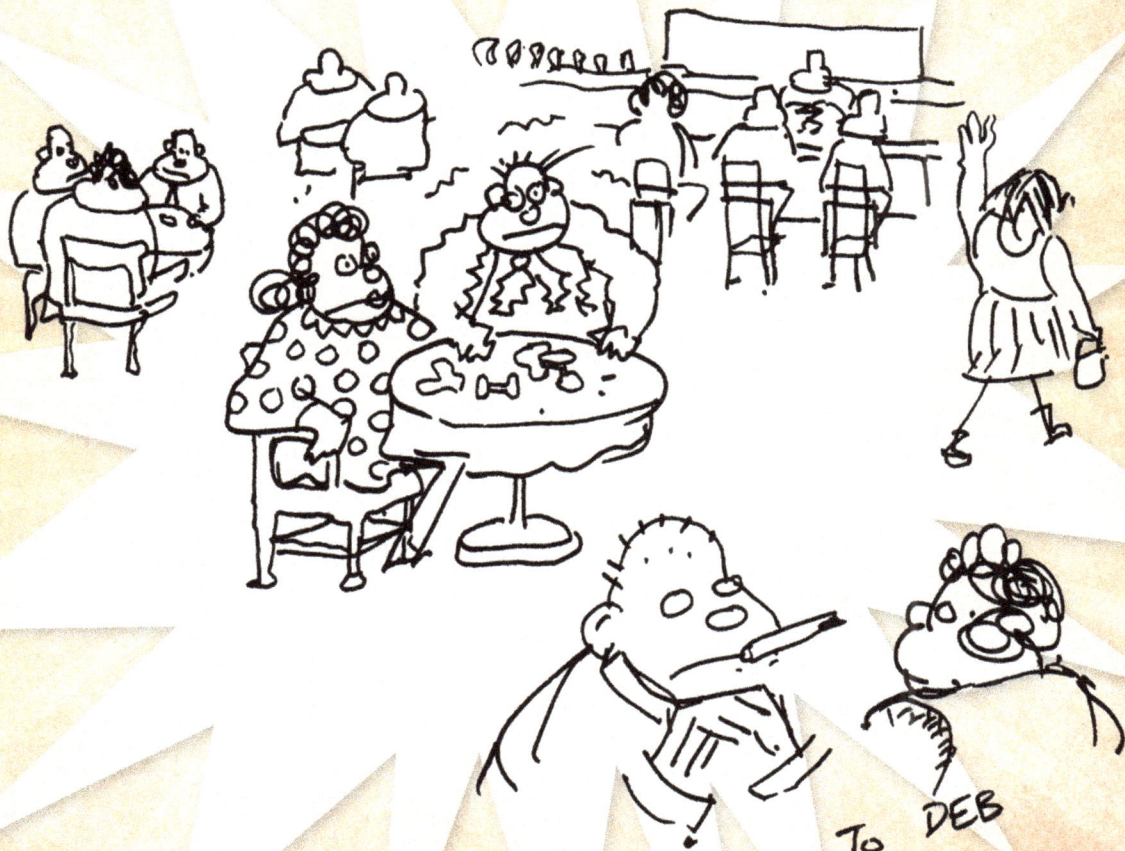

TO DEB

51

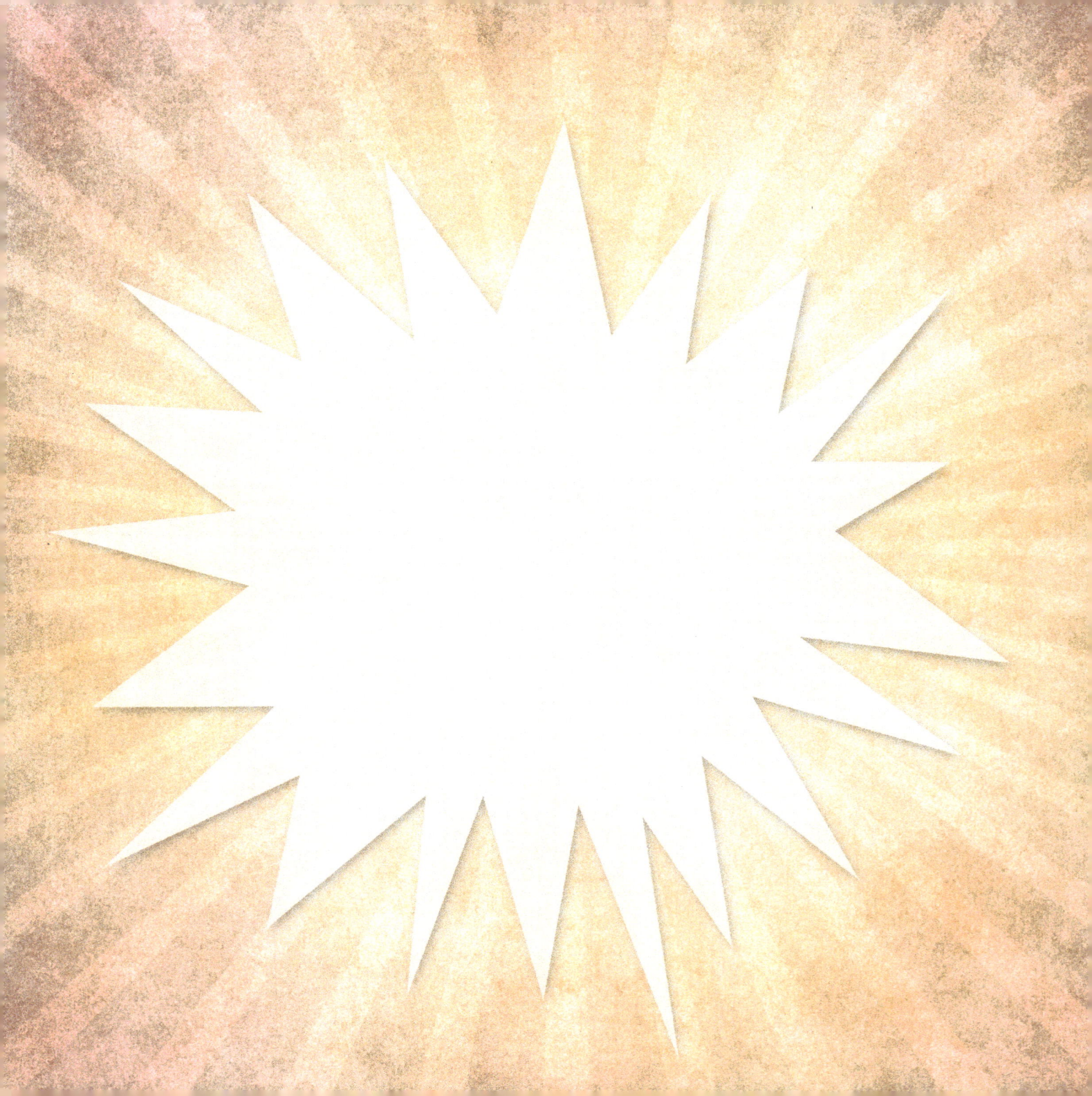

Story Jokes For The DIGNIFIED

HI! YOU TWO. WHERE YA GOING?

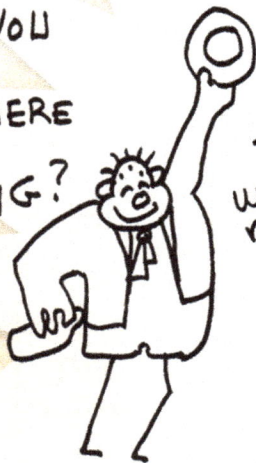

TO A MOZART CONCERT. TO HEAR THE C-MAJOR VIOLIN SONATA— WE UNDERSTAND THE FIRST MOVEMENT IS DISTINGUISHED BY IT'S LIGHT-FINGERED TEXTURE AND IT'S SIMPLICITY OF HARMONIC PATTERNS, WHILE THE 2ND CONTAINS SINUOUS MELODY THAT IS PROFOUNDLY PENSIVE. THE FINAL MOVEMENT, OF COURSE, REVERTS TO THE CAREFREE MOOD OF THE FIRST. WANT TO COME?

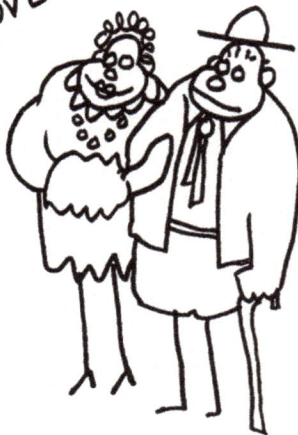

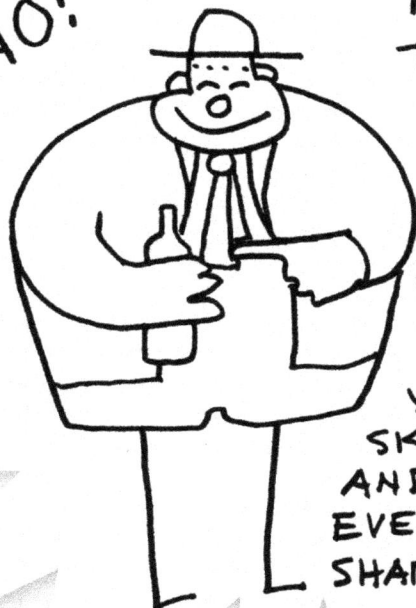

NO! IM GOING HOME TO SHAMPOO MY HAIR WITH PALMOLIVE! PERHAPS YOU'D RATHER SKIP THE CONCERT AND JOIN ME IN AN EVENING OF RICH SHAMPOO EXPERIENCE.

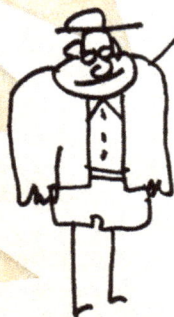
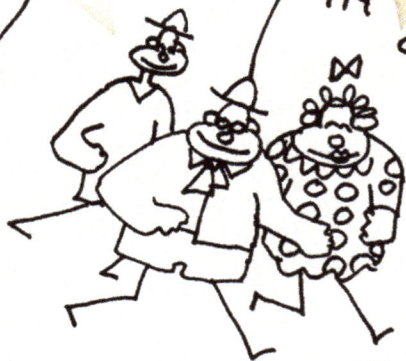
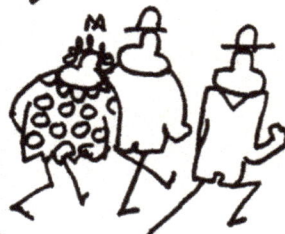
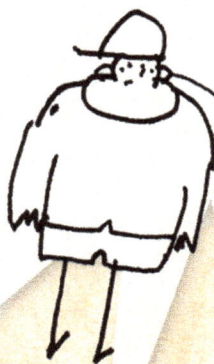

The Search

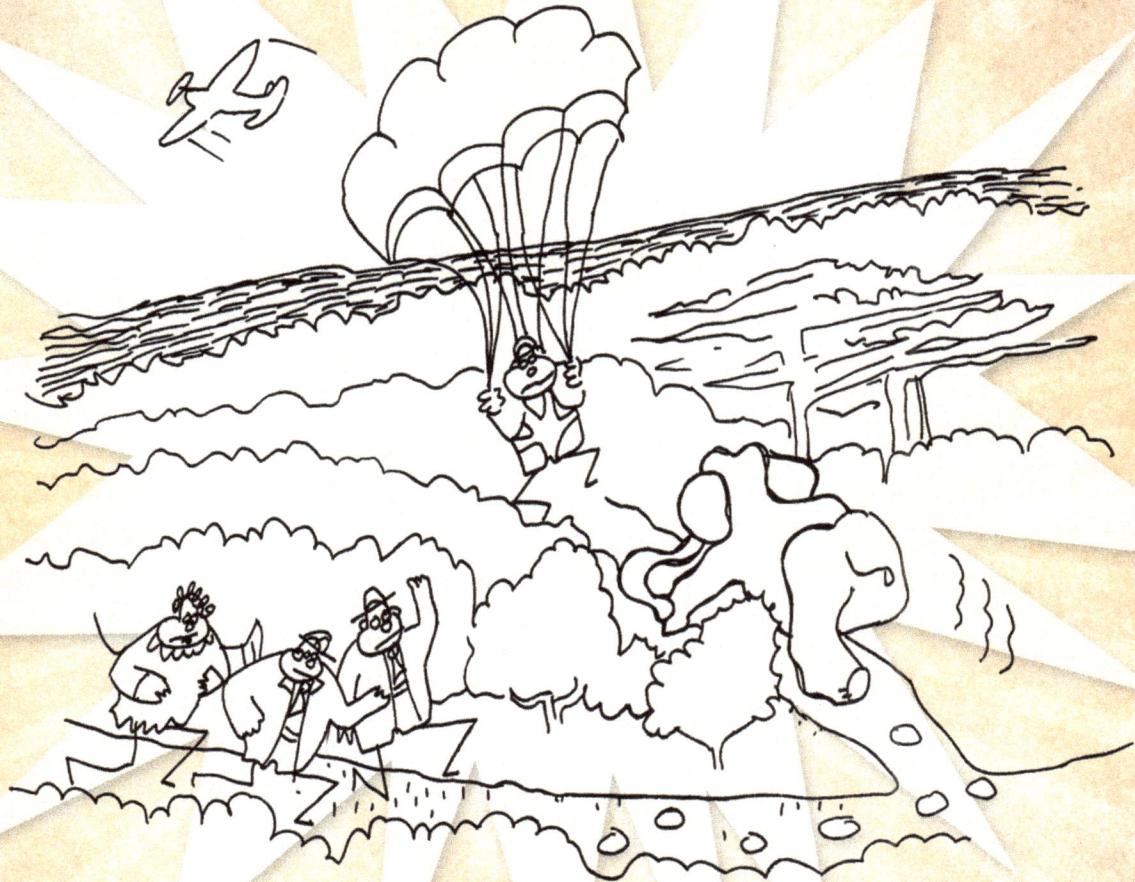

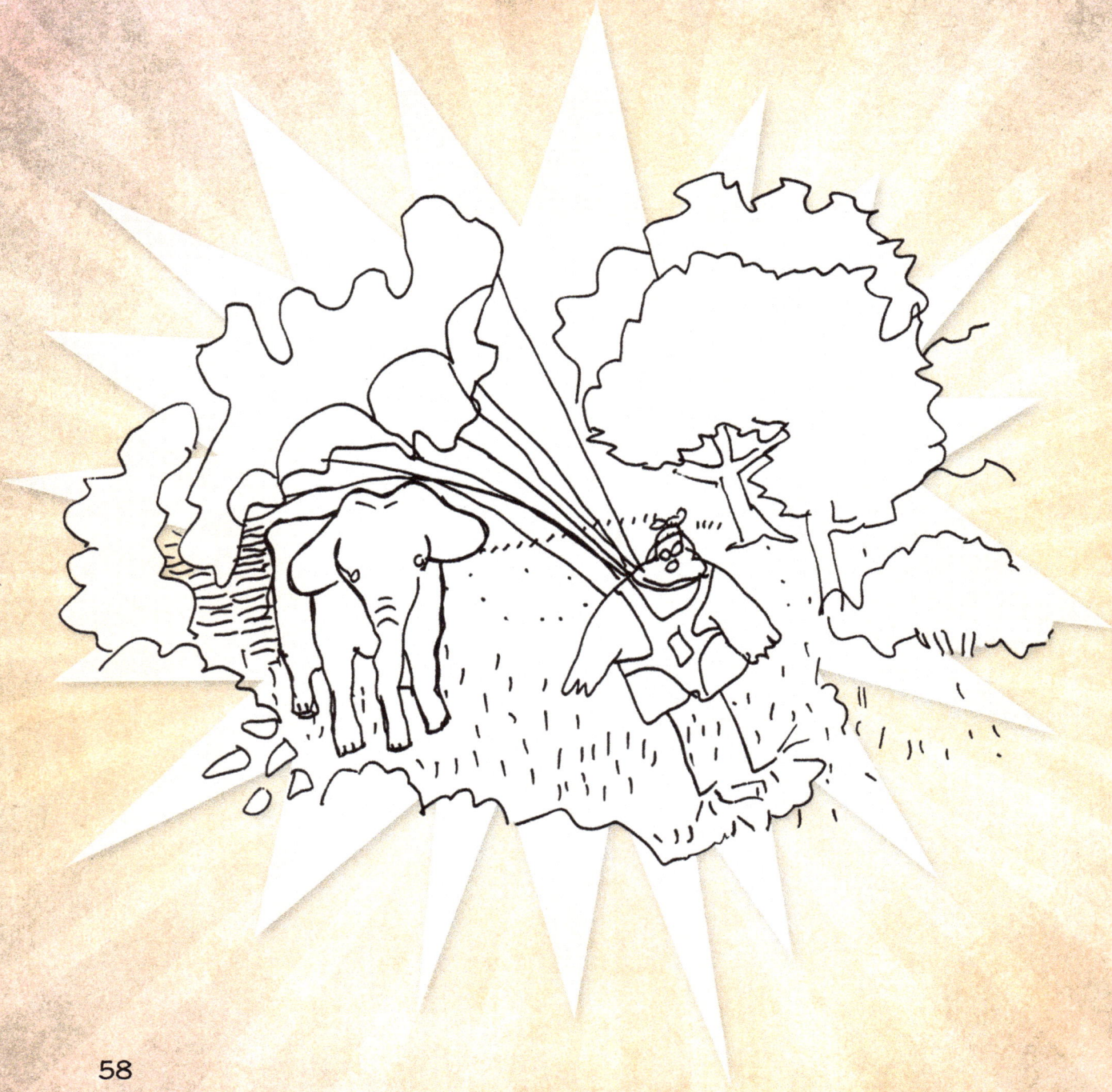

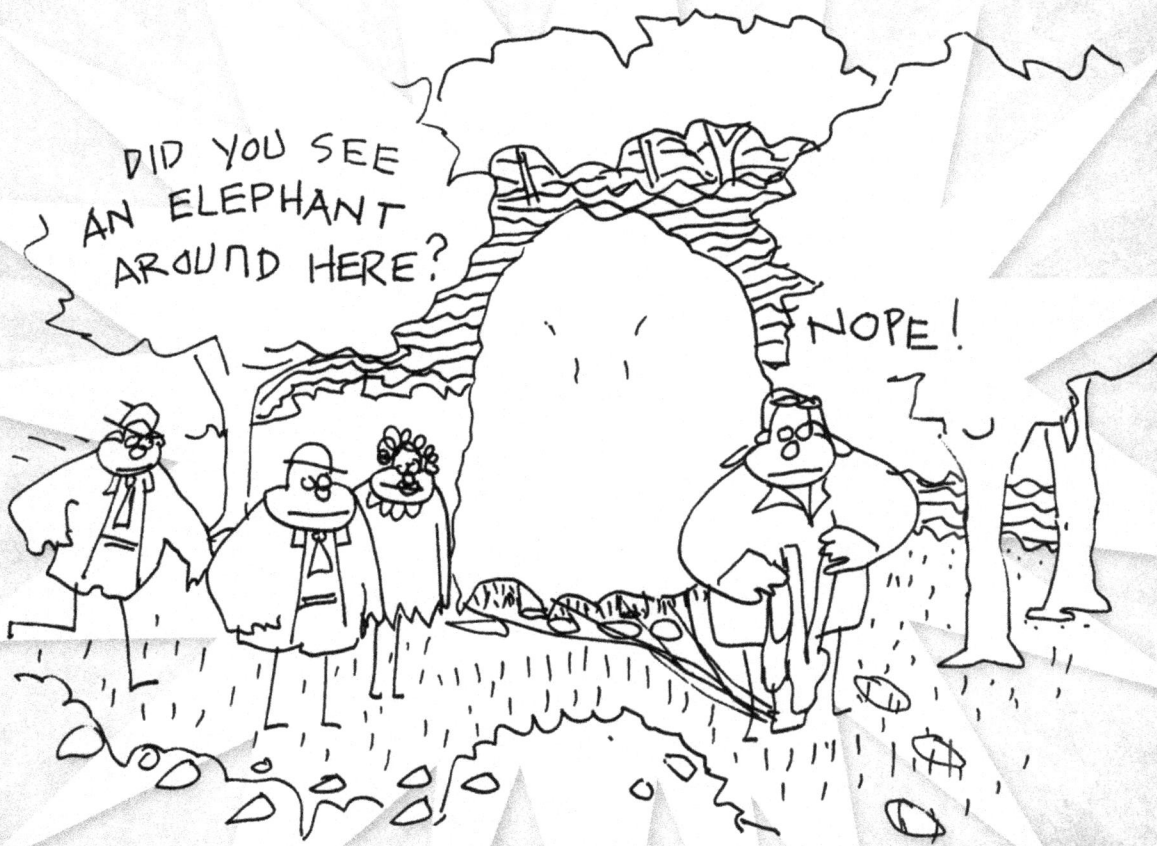

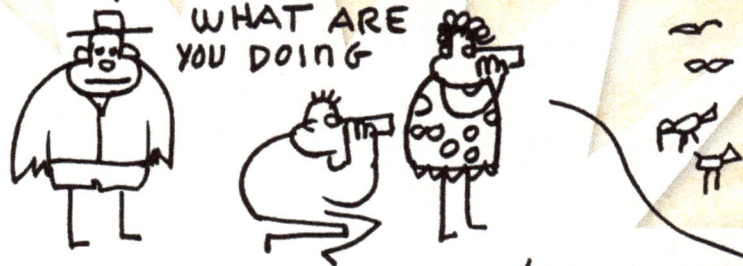

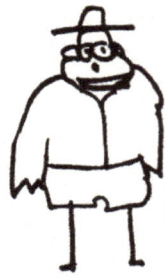

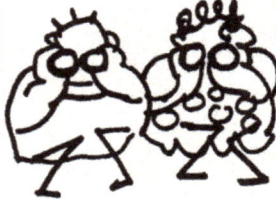

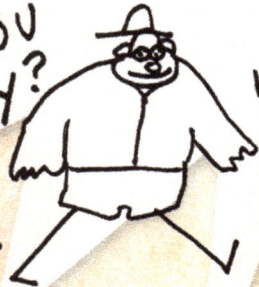

What's wrong with Hilda?

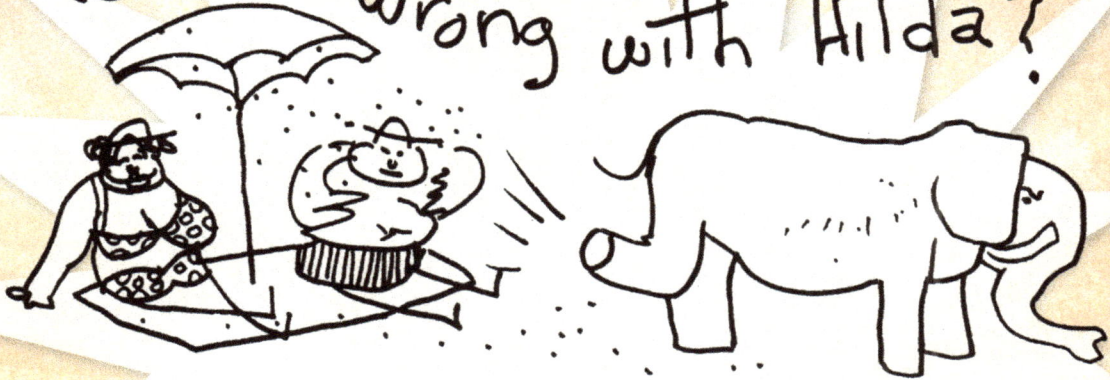

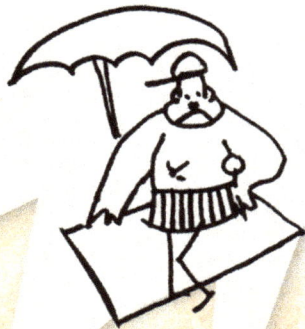

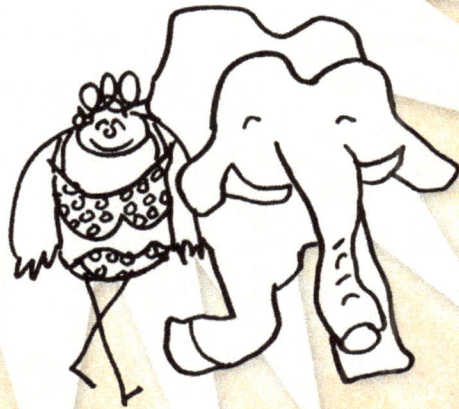

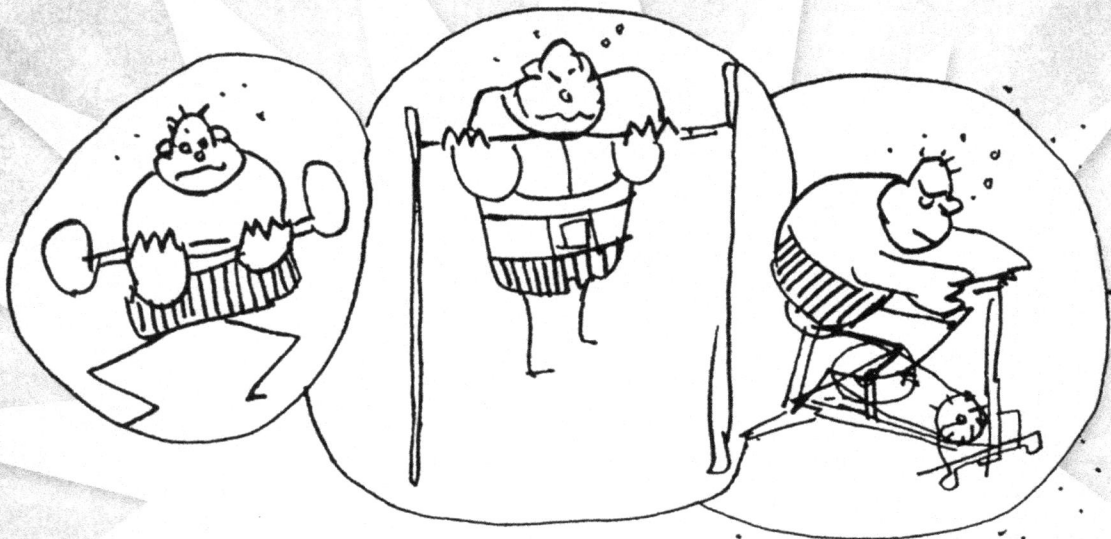

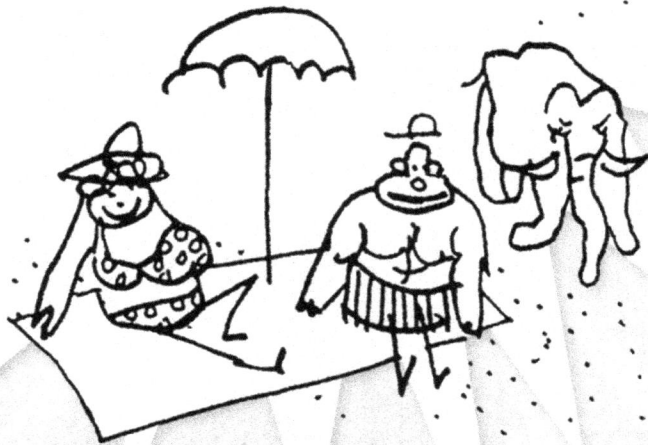

62

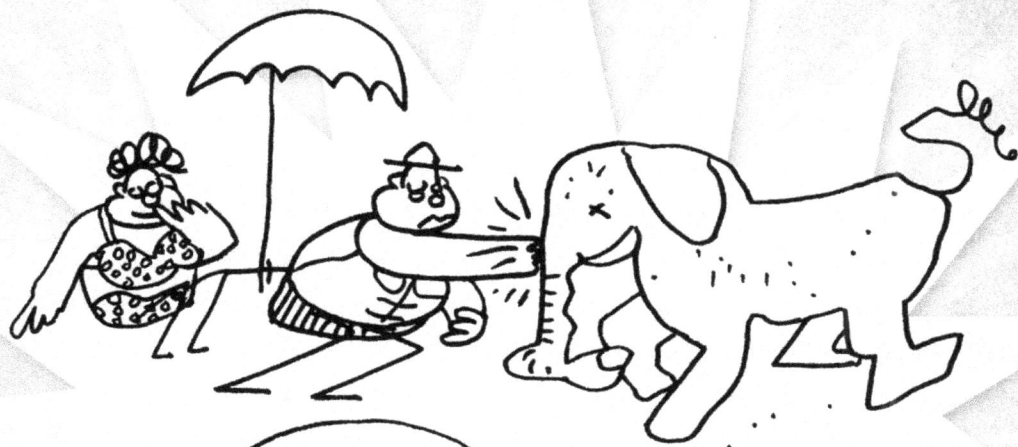

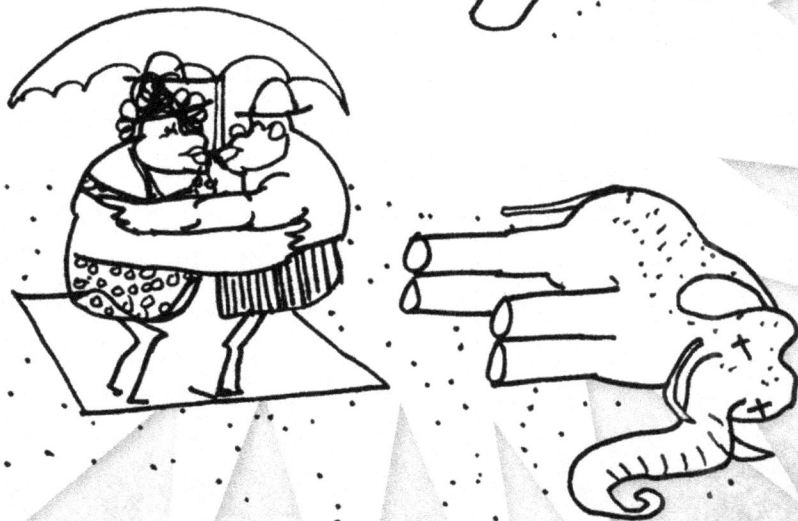

63

RORSCHACH TEST FOR DOGS.

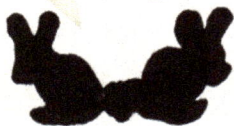

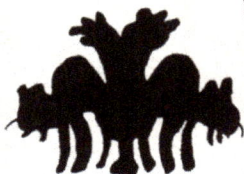

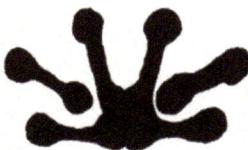

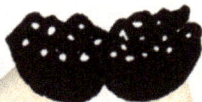

Spooner takes a Test.

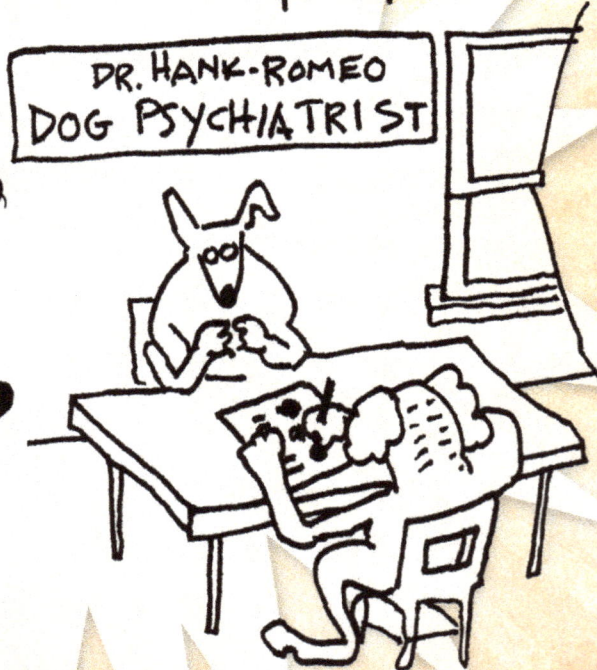

ELEPHANT ☑
TRAIN ☐
RABBITS ☐

ICEBERG ☐
CATS ☐
PIANO ☑

ENCYCLOPAEDIA ☑
CAMEL ☐
BONES ☐

DOG FOOD ☐
TANK ☐
MAILBOX ☑

DR. HANK-ROMEO
DOG PSYCHIATRIST

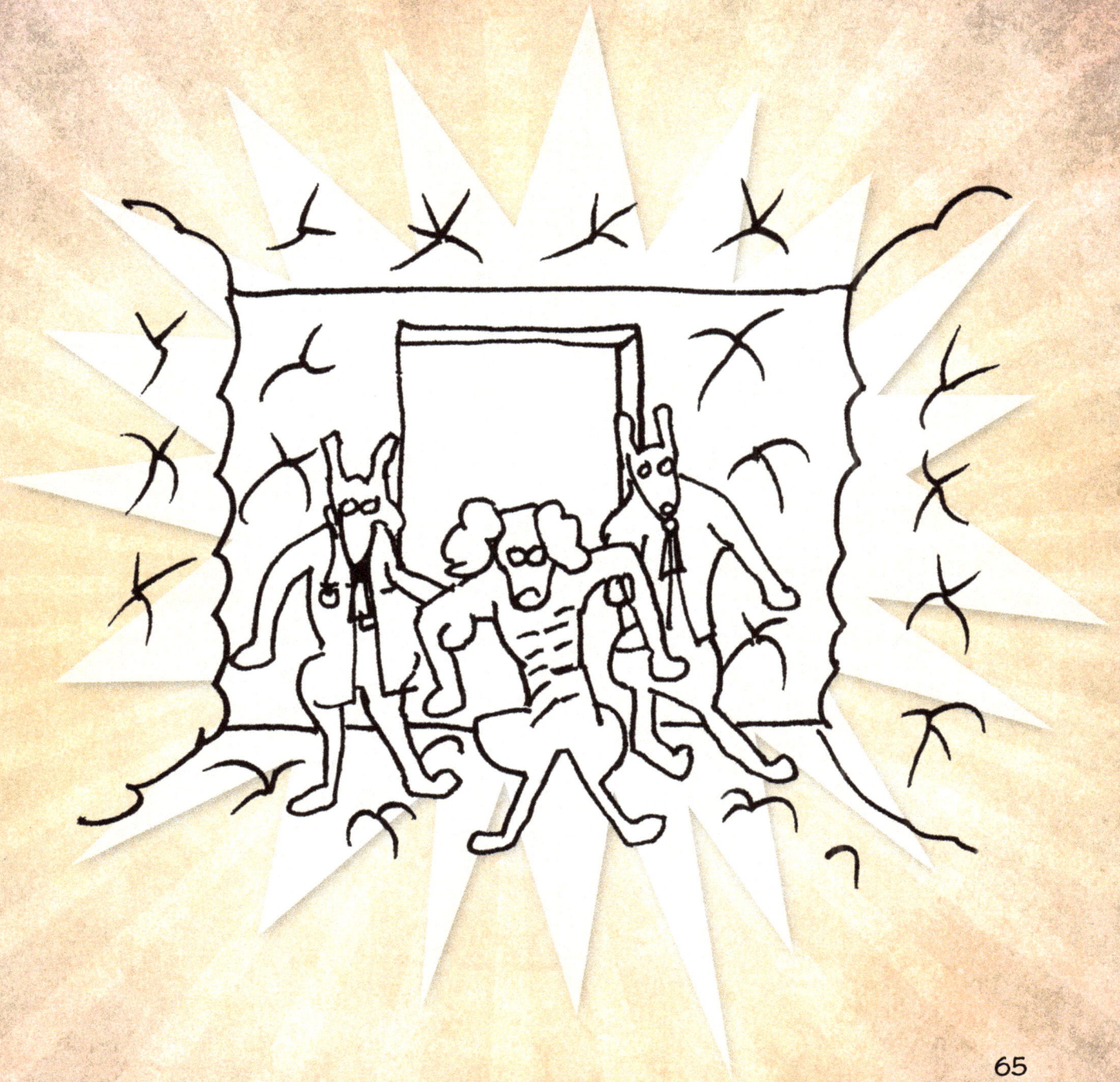

PASSION MAKES A PLEA.

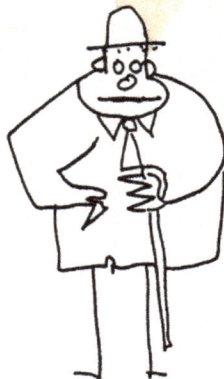

WHAT DO YOU DO?

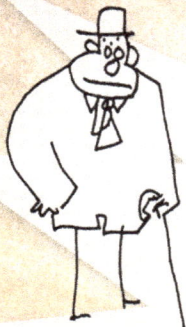

I WORK AT THE EXXON STATION. WHAT DO YOU DO?

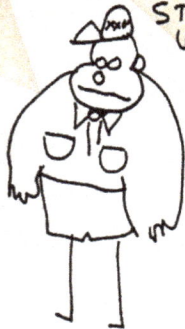

I'M PRESIDENT OF THE INTER-GALACTIC SPACE FELLOWSHIP TO FURTHER UNIVERSAL PEACE. WE'RE OFF, NOW, TO STOP THE IMPENDING WAR WHICH COULD RESULT THE IMPLOSION OF OUR GALAXY AND IT'S RETURN TO A "BLACK HOLE".

WANT TO COME?

NAW! I GOTTA GO WASH UP.

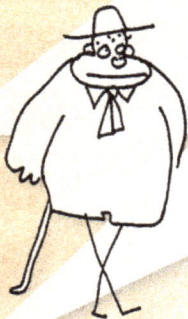

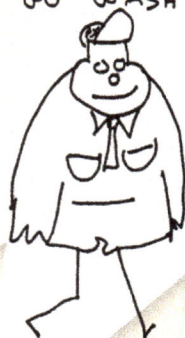

HISTORK INVENTION'S SERIES

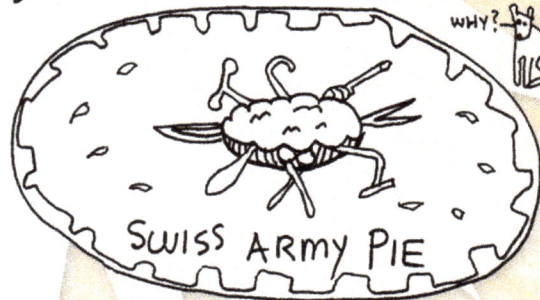

WHY?

SWISS ARMY PIE

66

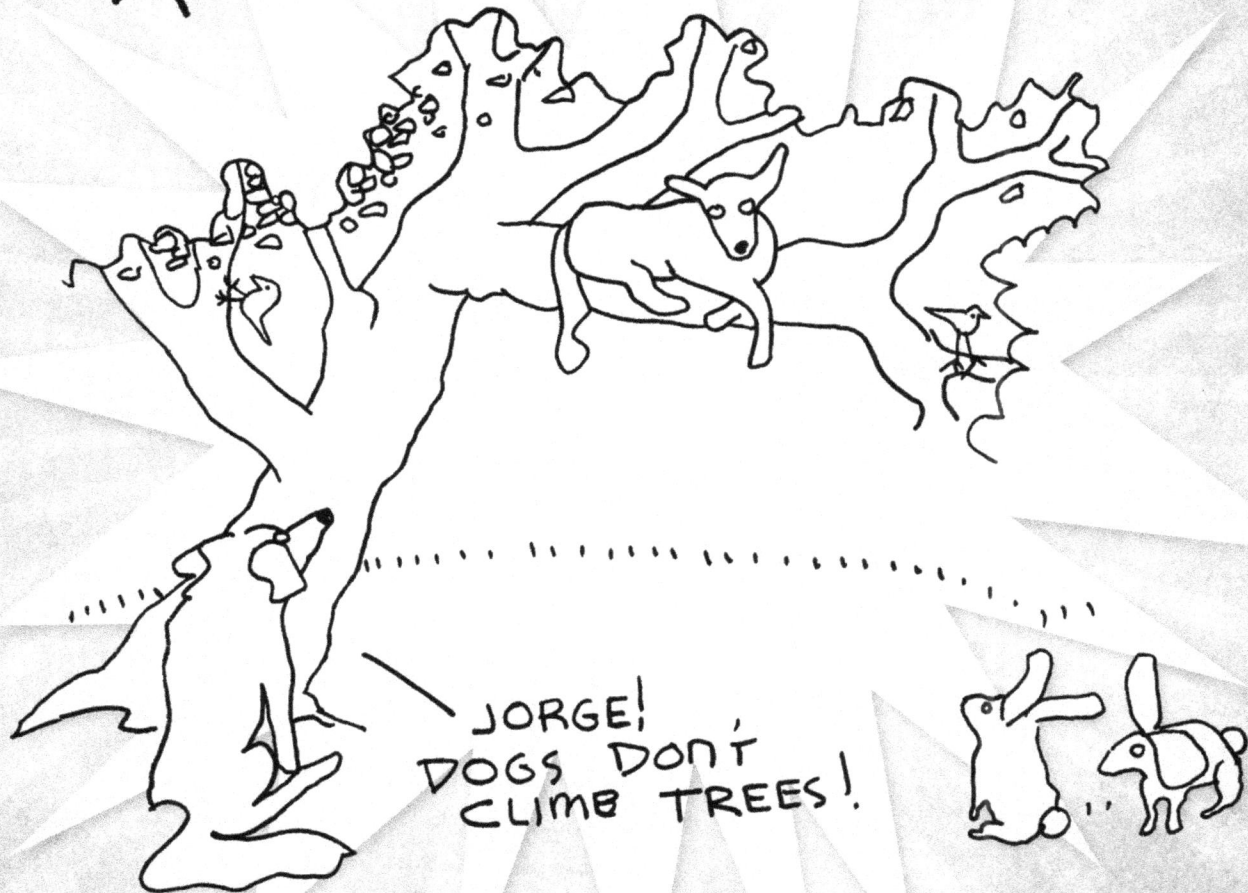

the Lesson.

JORGE! DOGS DON'T CLIMB TREES!

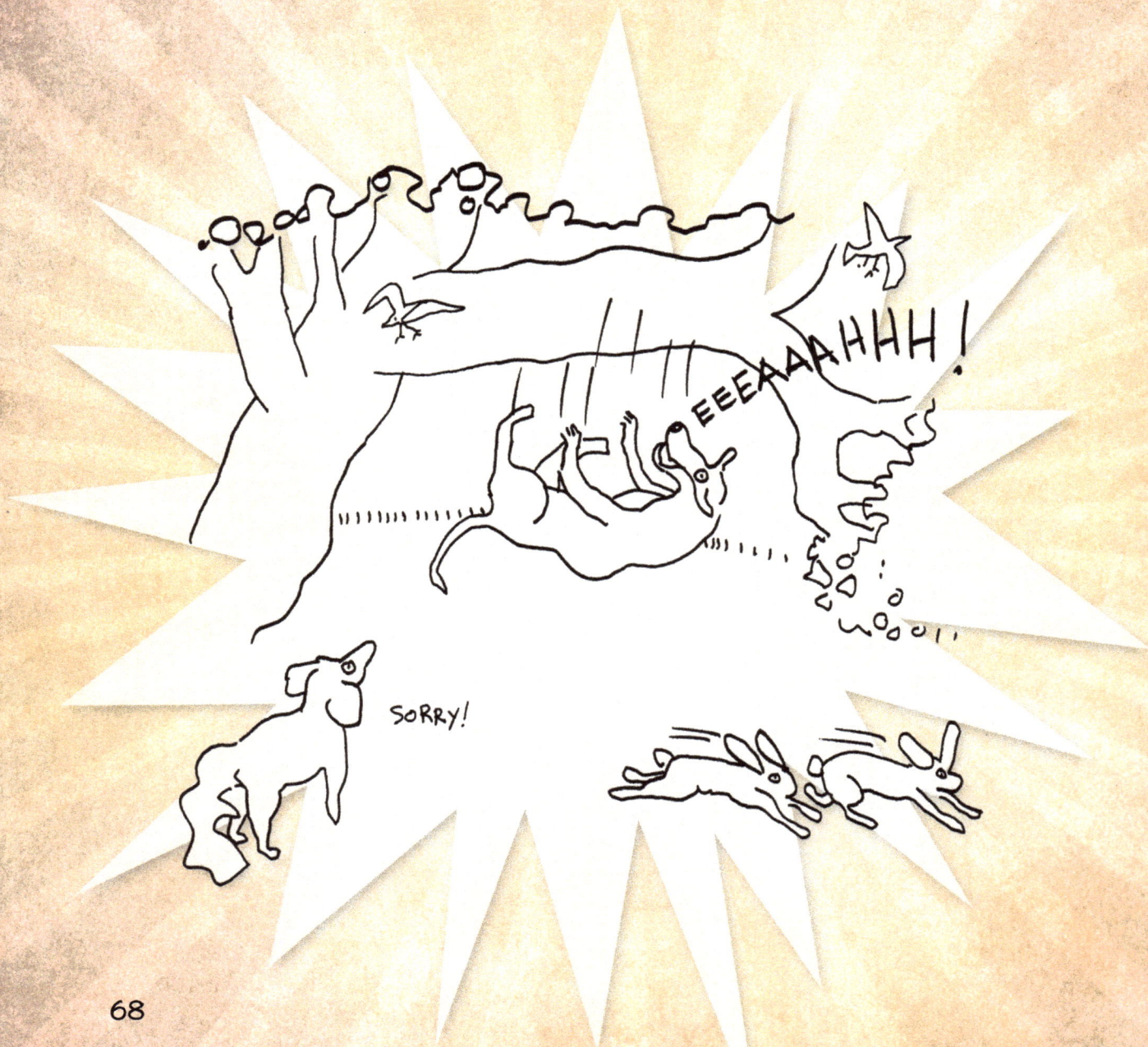

EEEAAAAHHH!

SORRY!

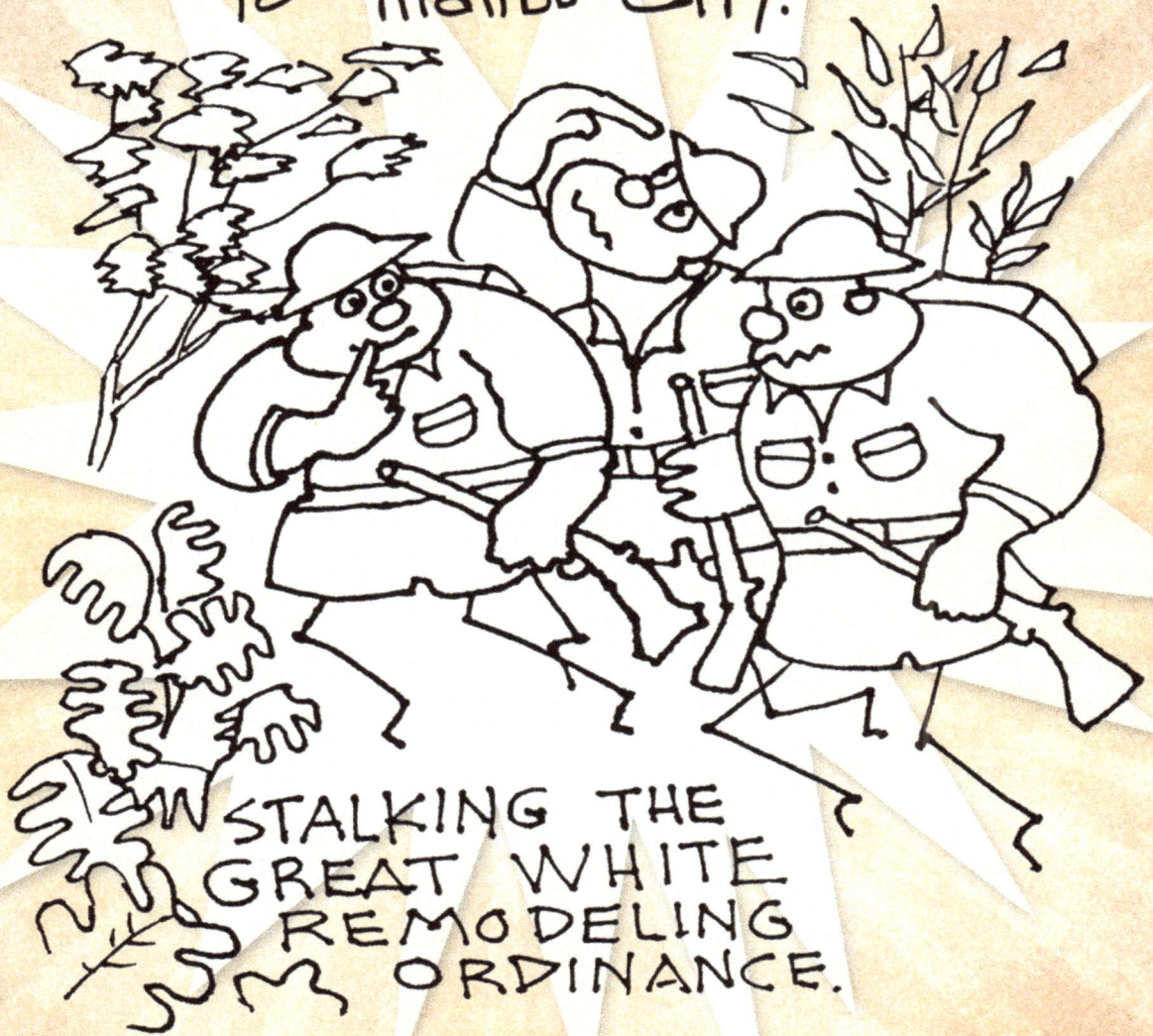

To Malibu City.

STALKING THE GREAT WHITE REMODELING ORDINANCE.

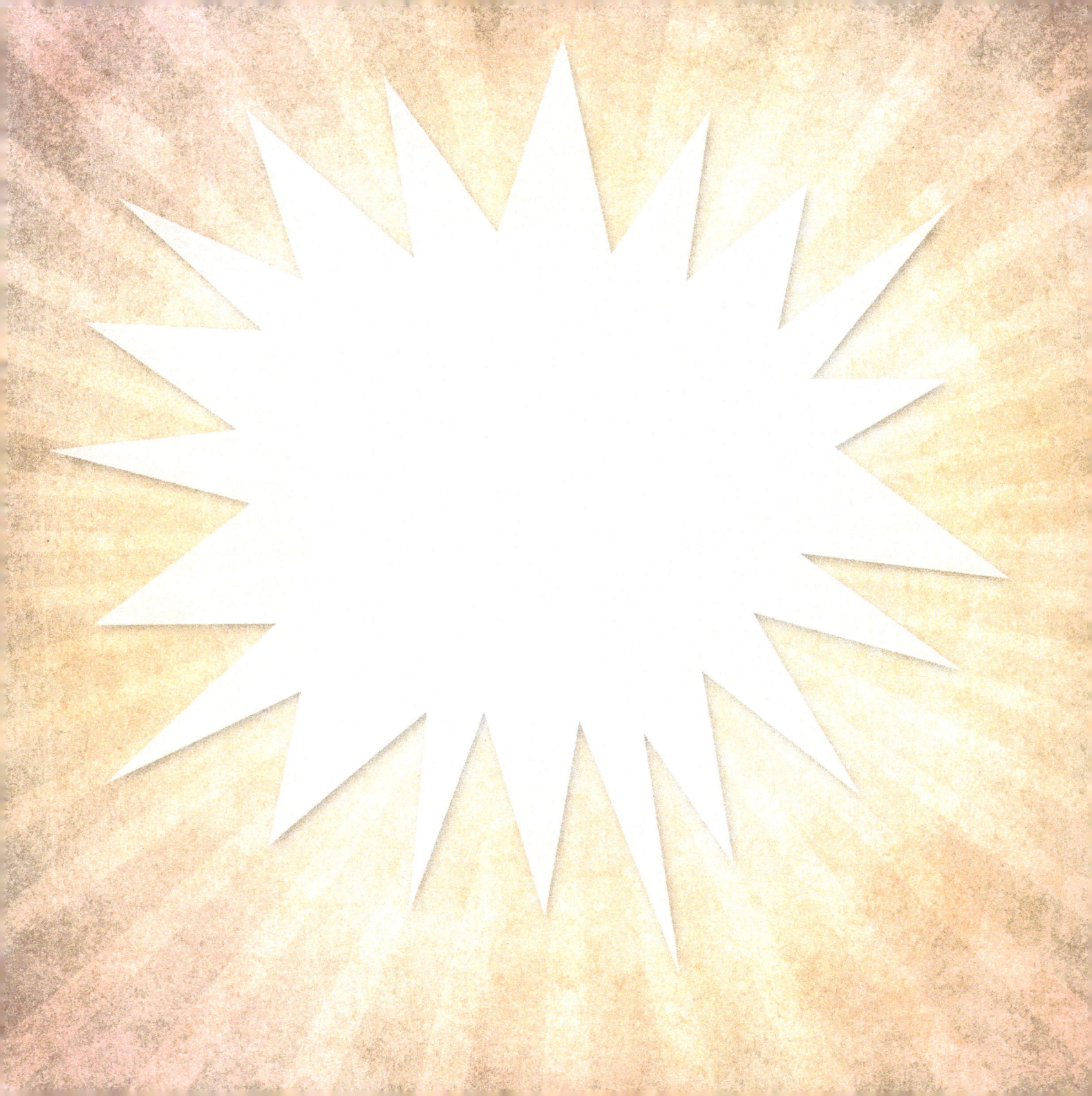

DETECTIVE FRED
IN
The Great Cow Mystery.

STARRING: (IN ORDER OF OCCURENCE)

FRED Helen
Patsy and BESSIE

IM DETECTIVE
FRED

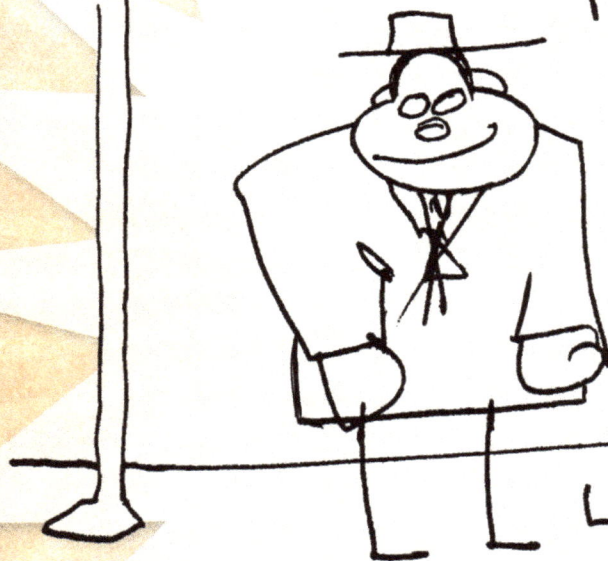

I FIND LOST PERSONS, SOLVE CRIMES TAIL PEOPLE LEAP OUT SUDDENLY FROM THE BUSHES. THINGS LIKE THAT.

72

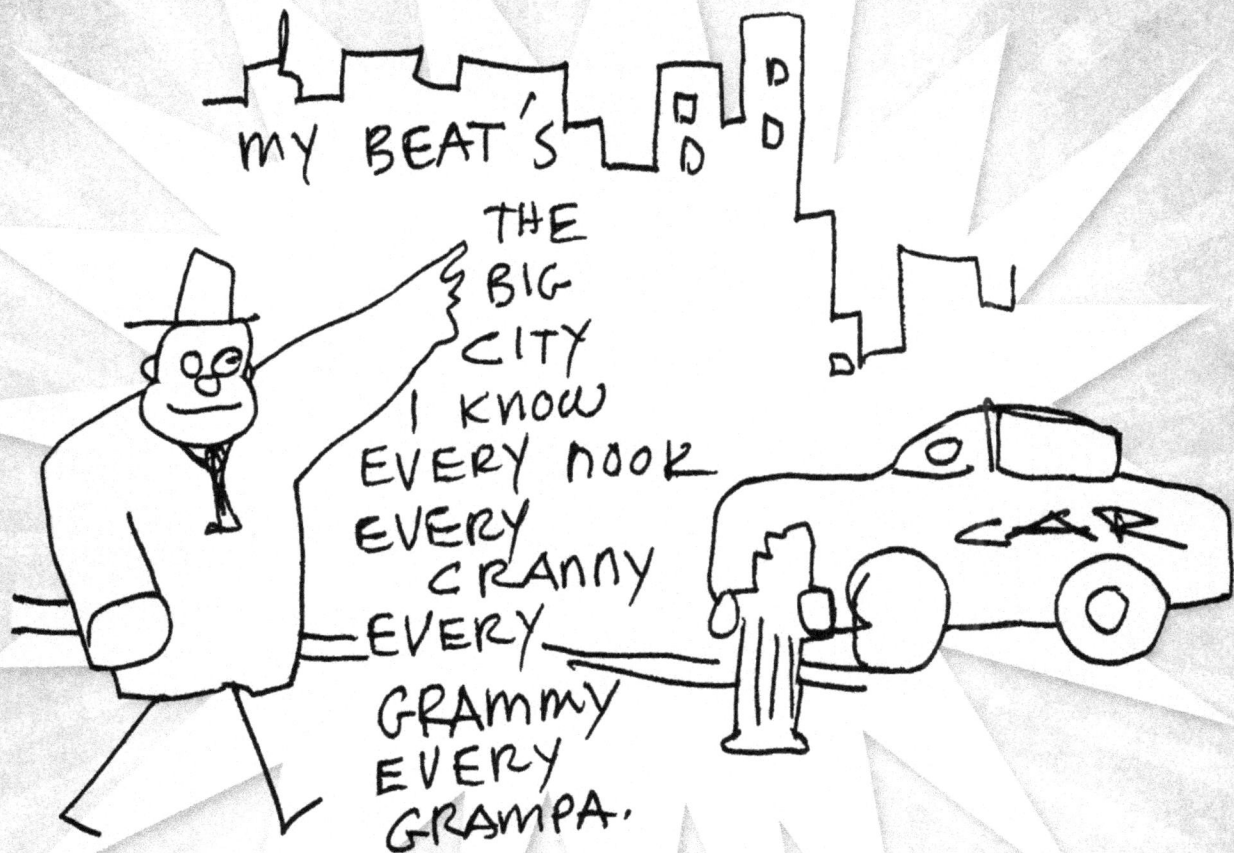

MY BEAT'S THE BIG CITY I KNOW EVERY NOOK EVERY CRANNY EVERY GRAMMY EVERY GRAMPA.

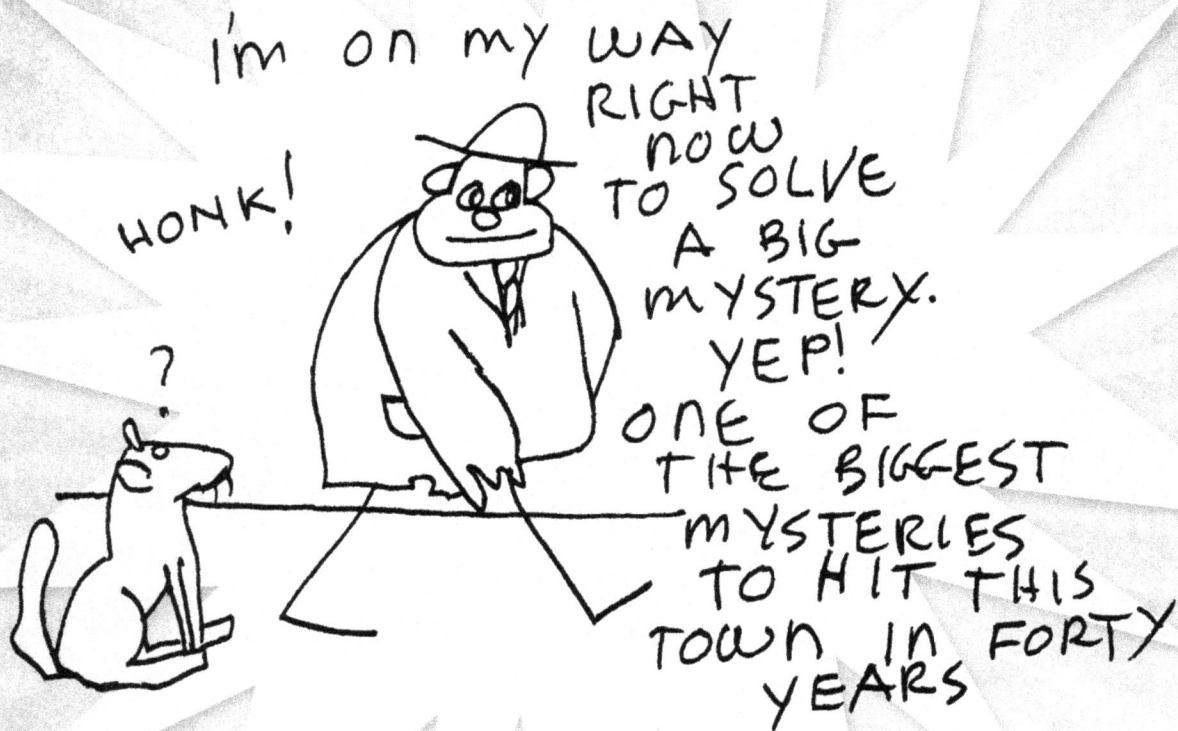

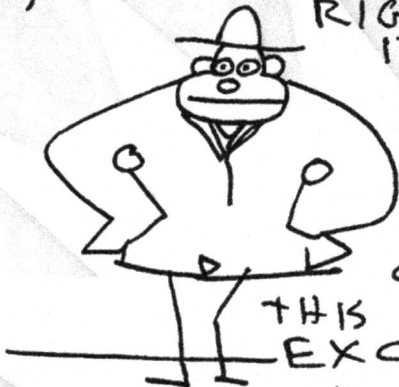

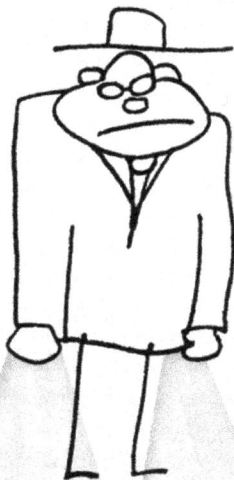

HERE!
I'LL JUST
GET
MY
EASLE
OUT
OF THIS
CAR AND
DRAW YOU
A PICTURE
OF HER.

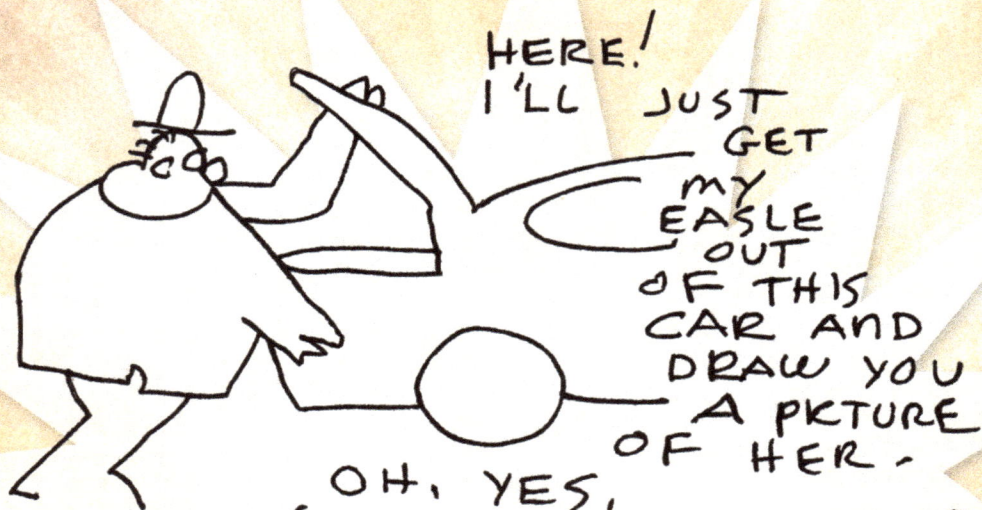

OH, YES,
I'M AN
ARTIST,
TOO,
STUDIED
AT
THE
ACADAMEY
I'M NOT
MUCH OF A
SPELLER
THOUGH,

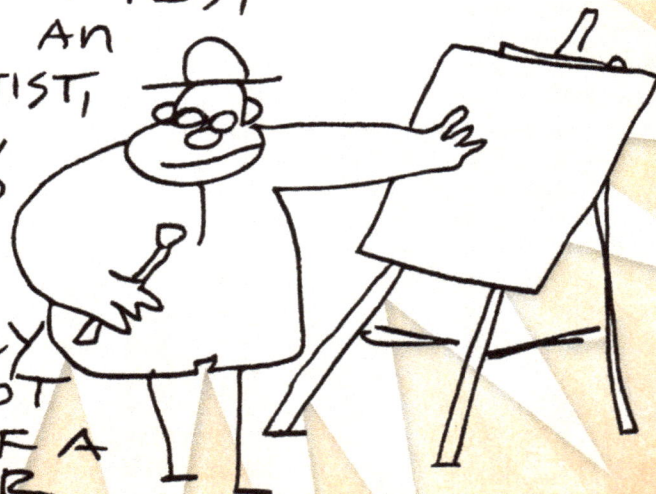

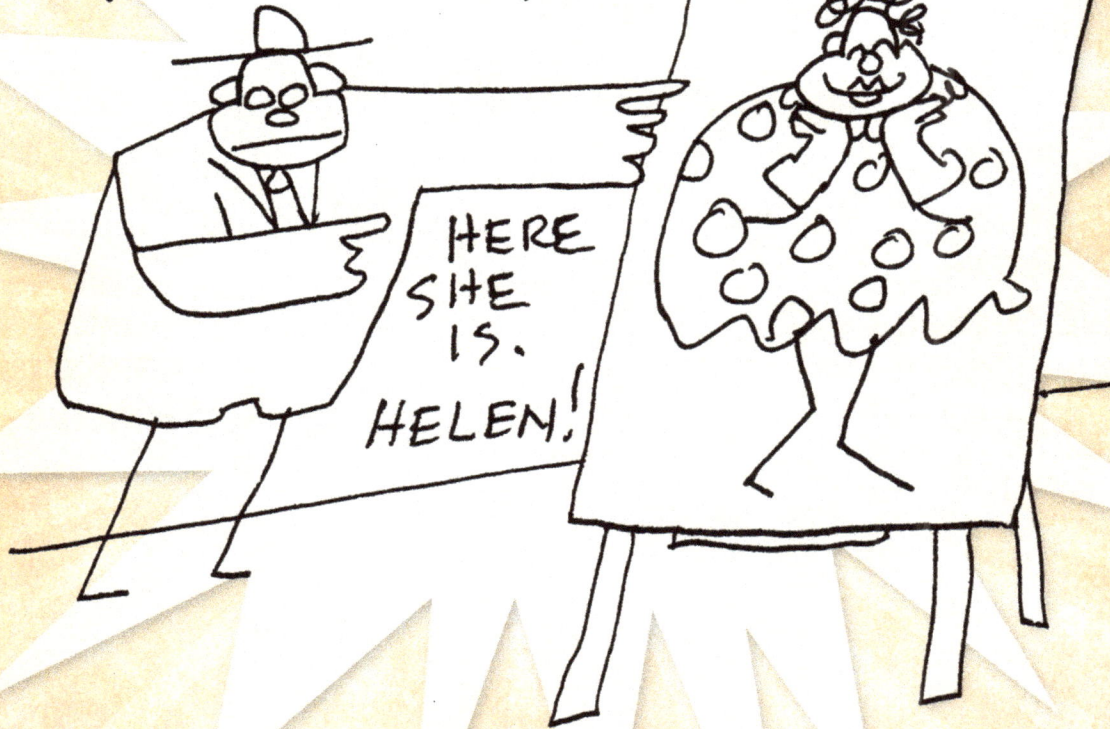

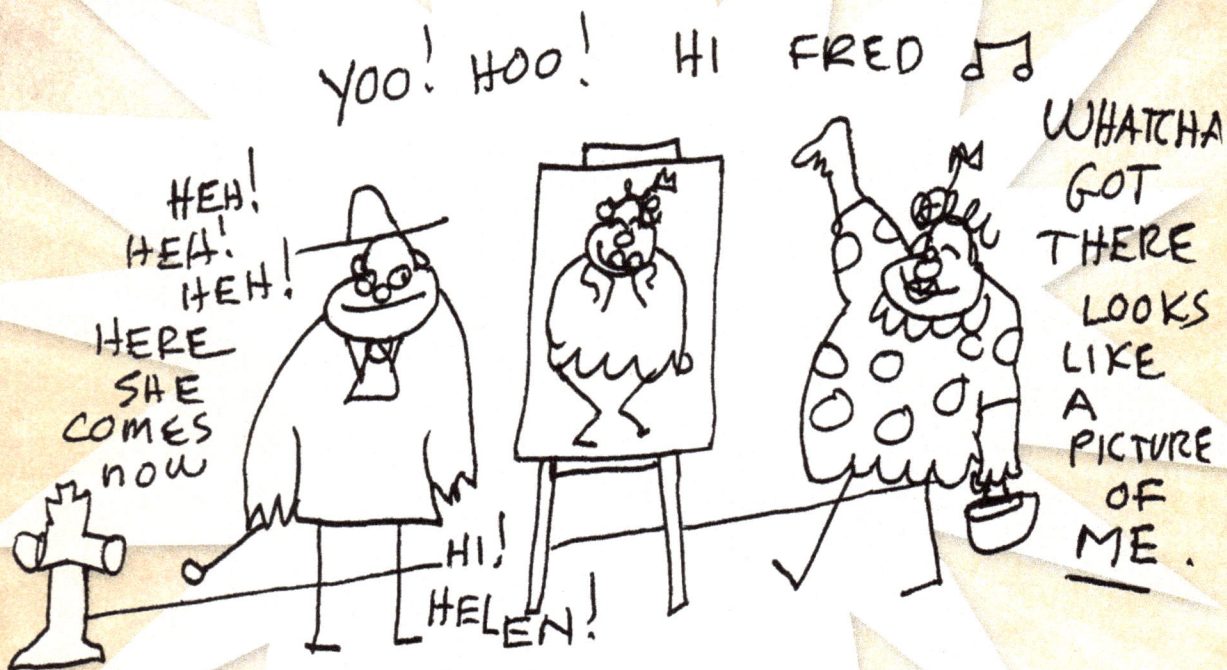

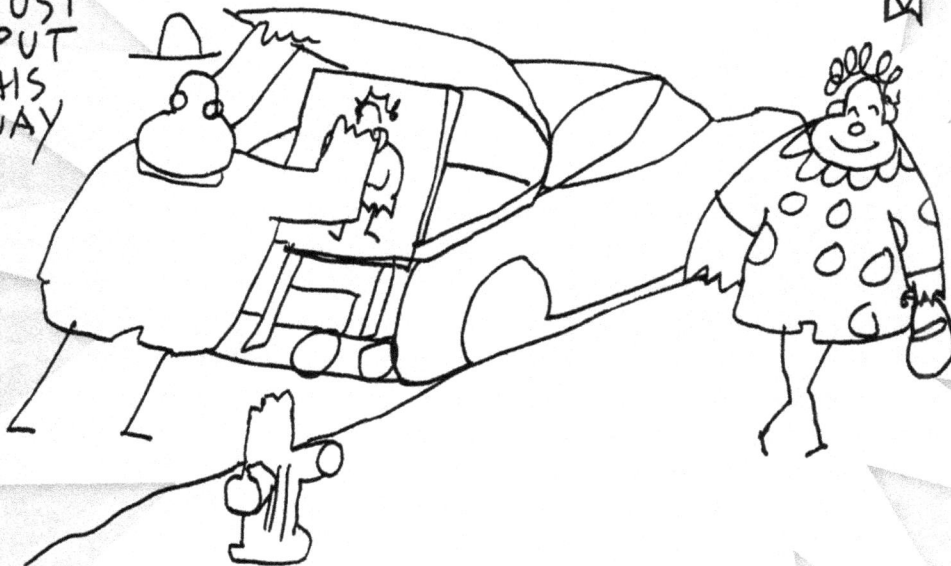

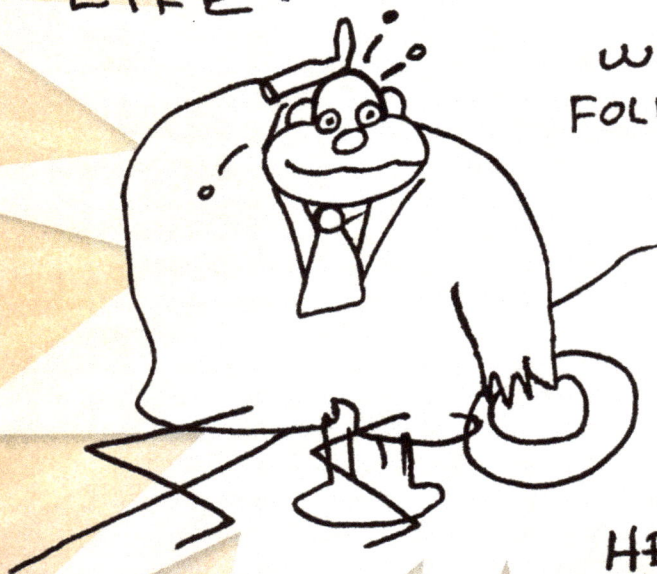

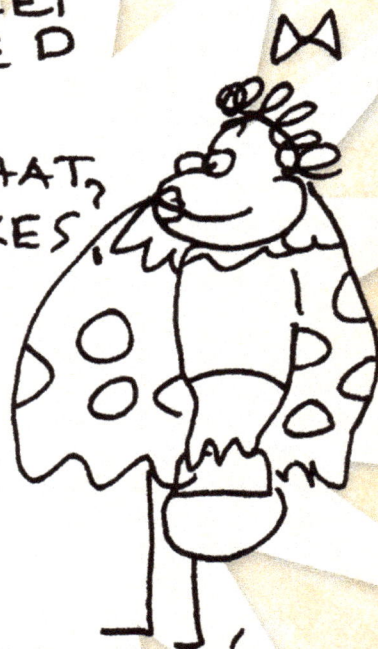

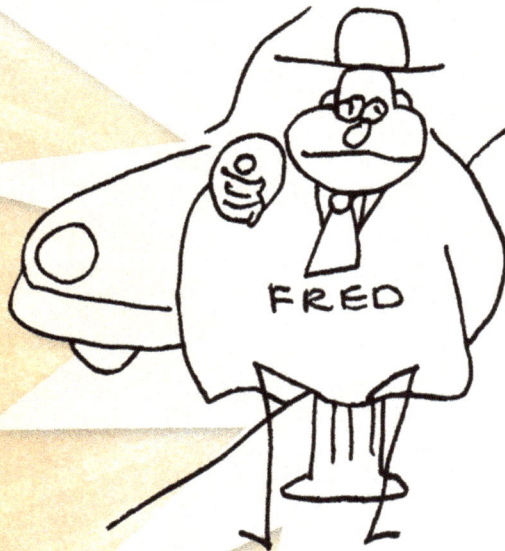

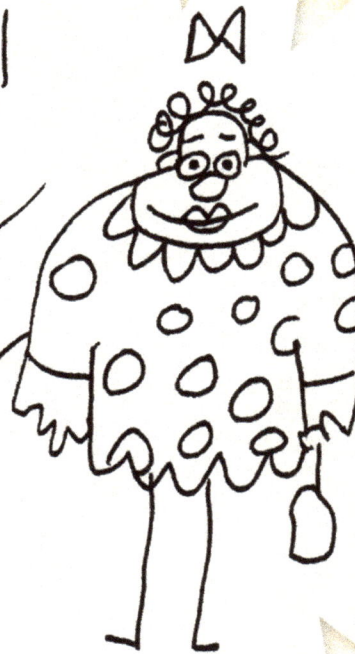

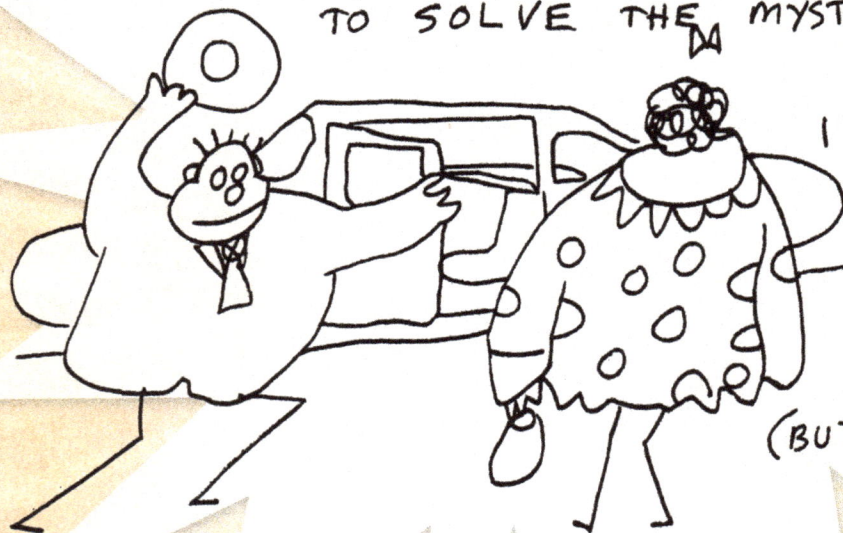

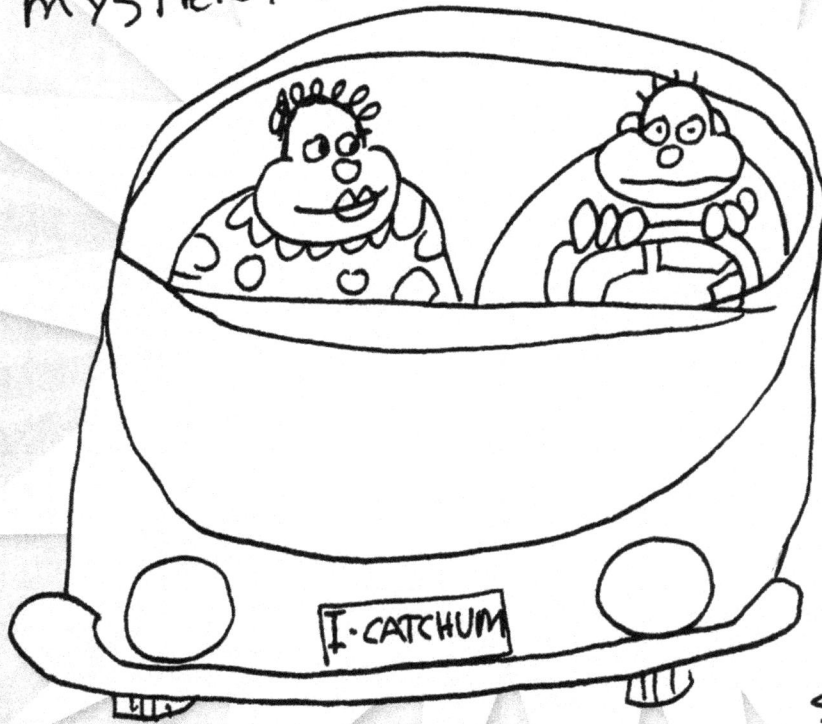

WHAT IS THE BIG MYSTERY, FRED?

YOU MEAN YOU FORGOT? BOY! HAVE YOU GOT A SHORT MEMORY. YOUR PET COW HAS BEEN MISSING SINCE SATURDAY.

I. CATCHUM

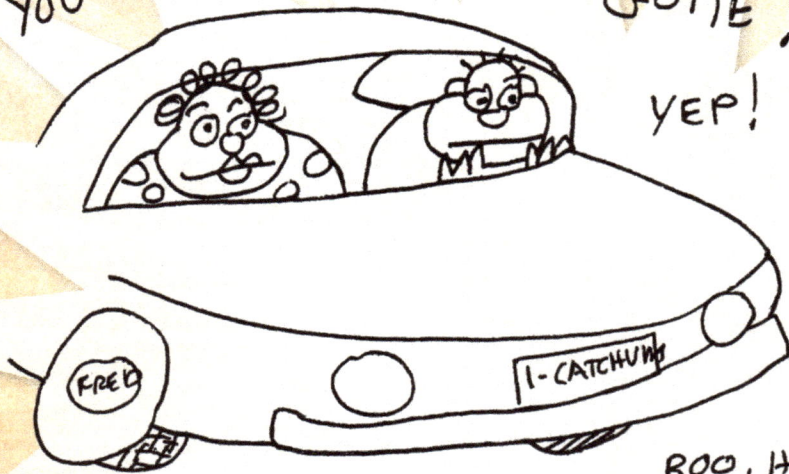
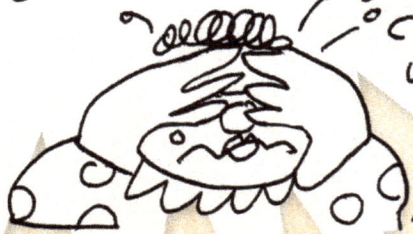

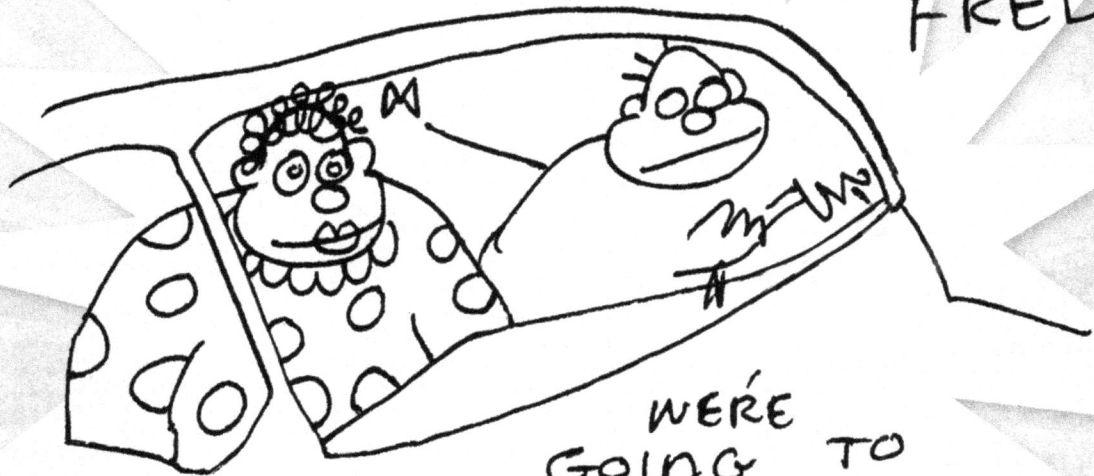

WUBBA, WEEBA, GOMNA, DO-A NOW, FRED?

WE'RE GOING TO THE PASTURE WHERE SHE WAS LAST SEEN. — PATSIE'S PASTURE THAT IS.

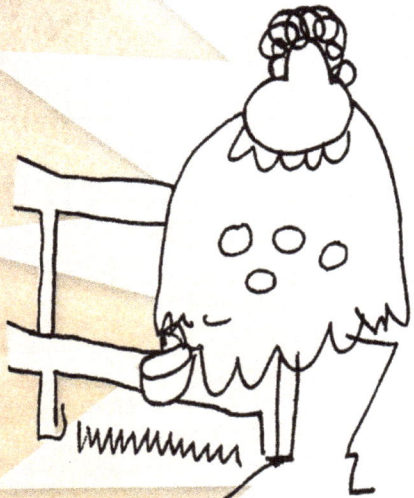
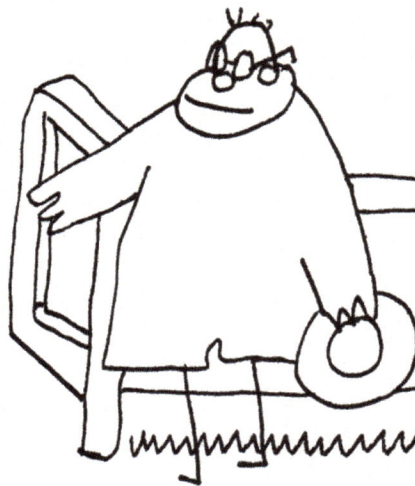
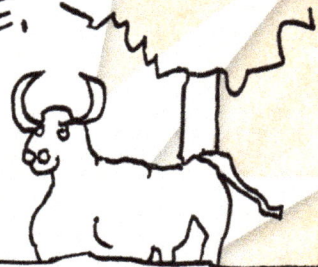

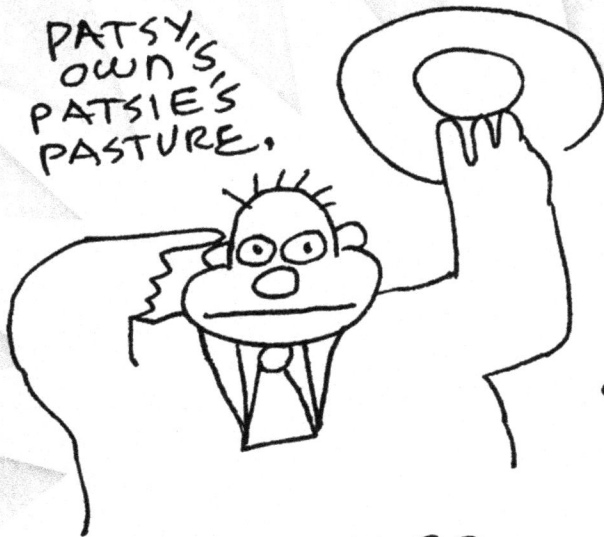

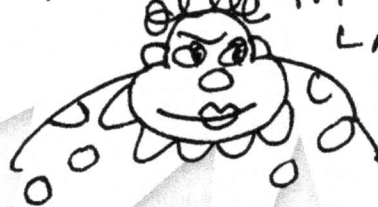

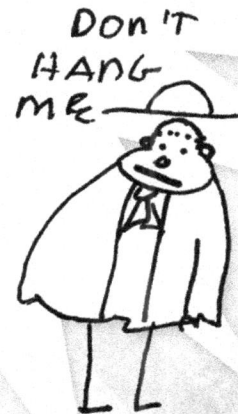

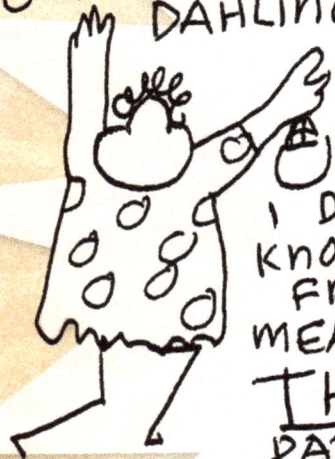
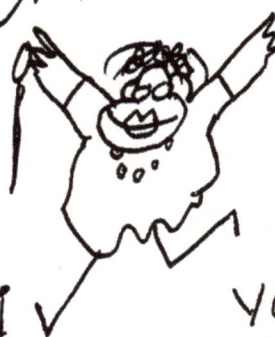

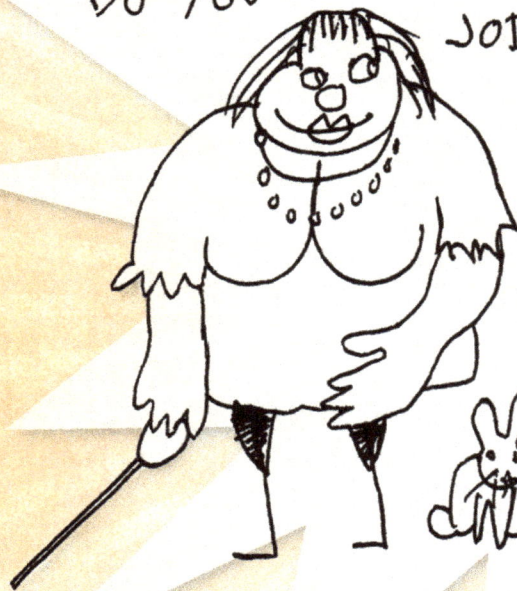
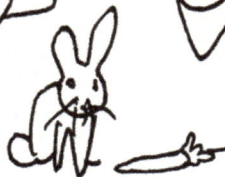
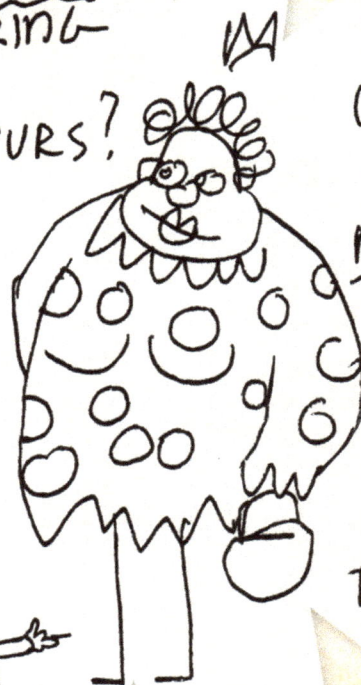

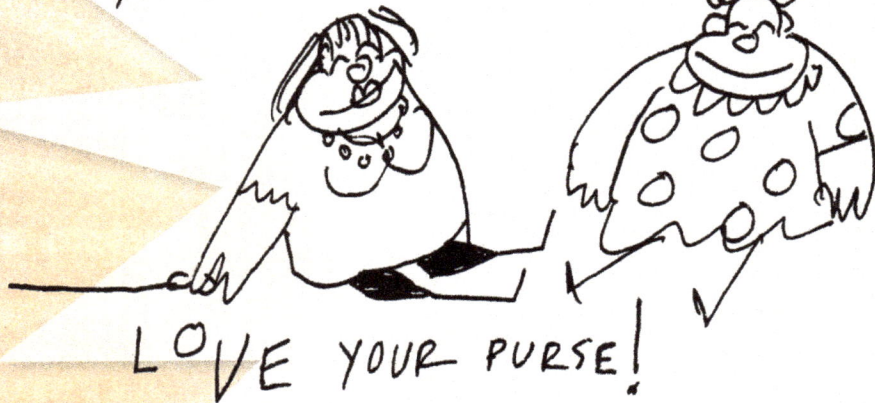

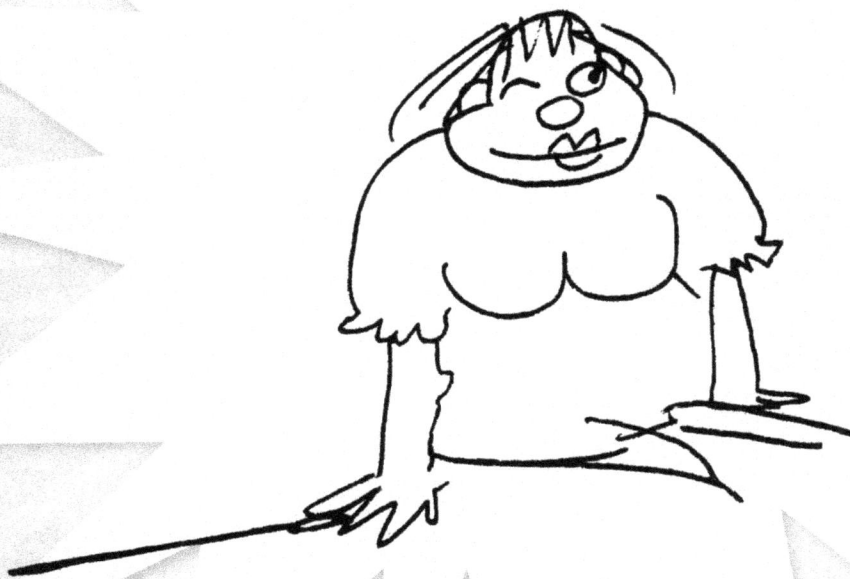

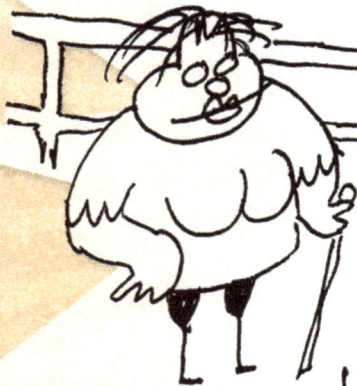

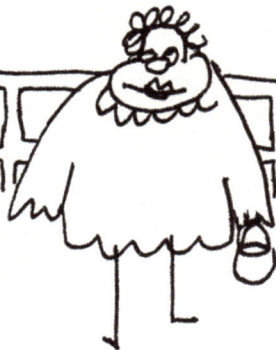

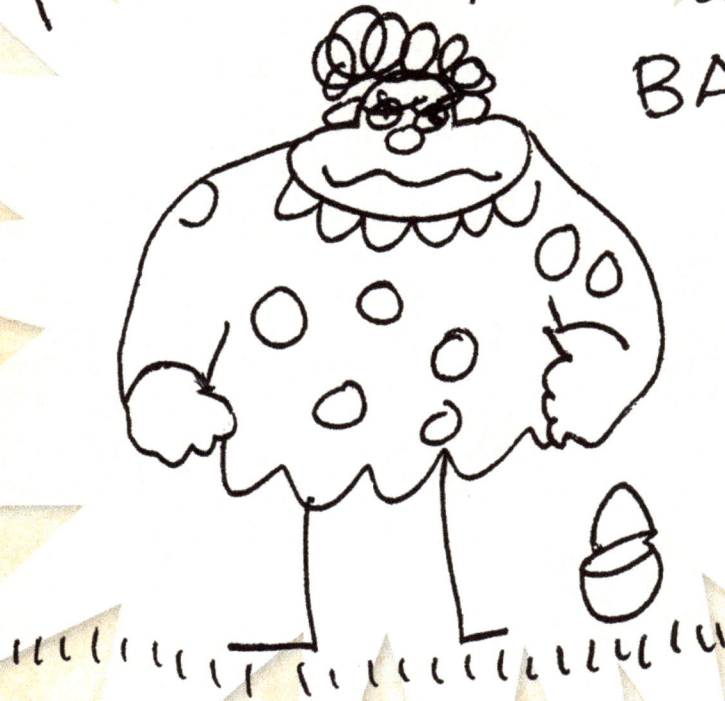

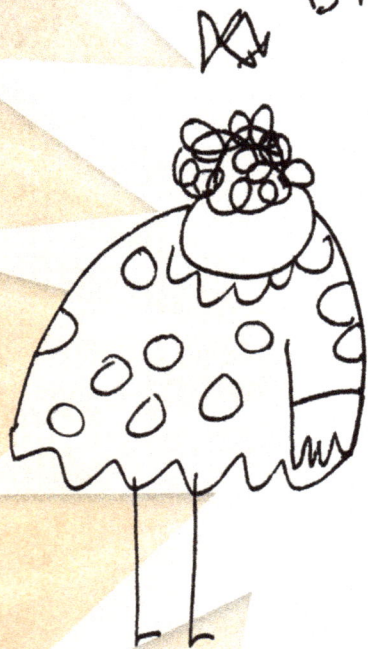
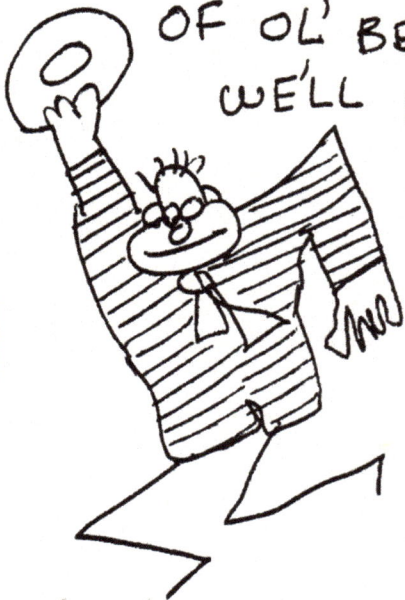

94

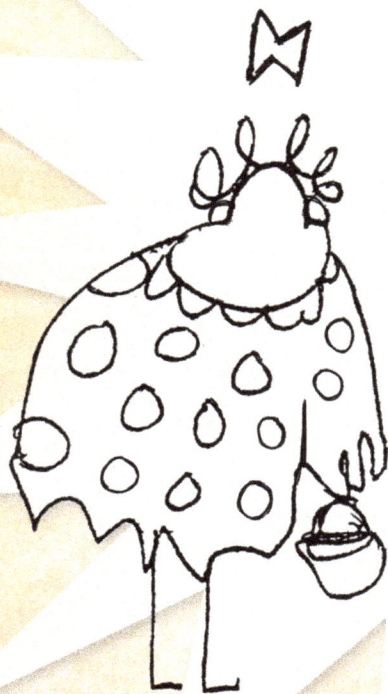

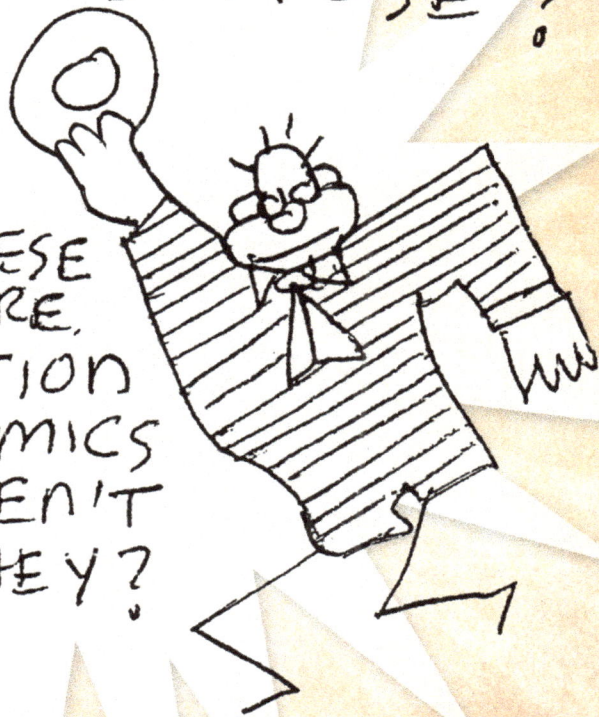

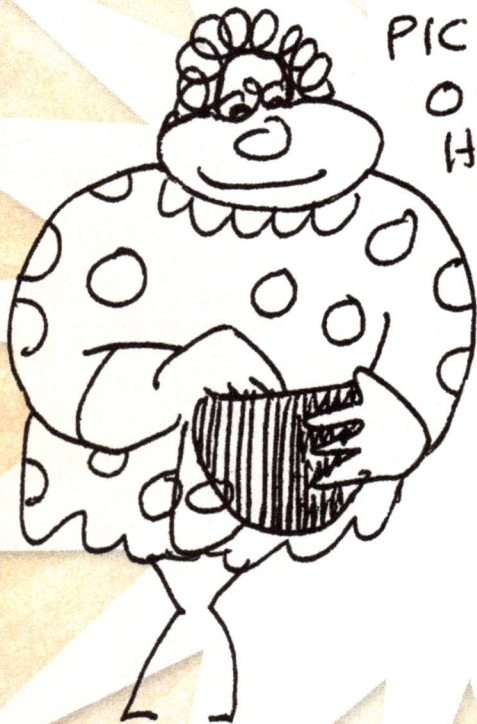

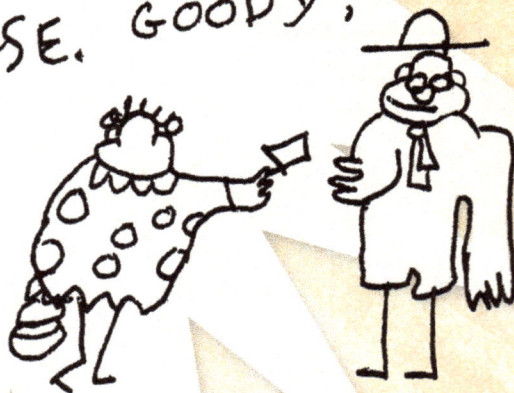

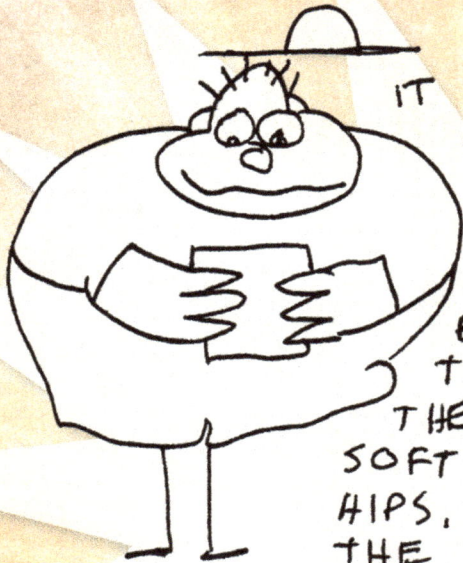

IT WAS HER ALL RIGHT. THE FOUR LEGS, THE WHITE BODY WITH LARGE BROWN PATCHES, THE SOULFUL EYES, THE CLOVEN HOOFS, THE SOFT MUZZLE, THE SQUARE HIPS, THE LARGE FRAME, THE UDDER, THE DULL-EYED STARE, ETC. ETC. BESSY REMINDED ME OF SOMEONE. I COULDN'T THINK WHO. AN OLD GIRL FRIEND? NO! I DON'T HAVE ANY OLD GIRL FRIENDS! MY MOTHER? NO, THE COLORING ISN'T RIGHT. ITS A BLACK AND WHITE PICTURE.

HMMM!

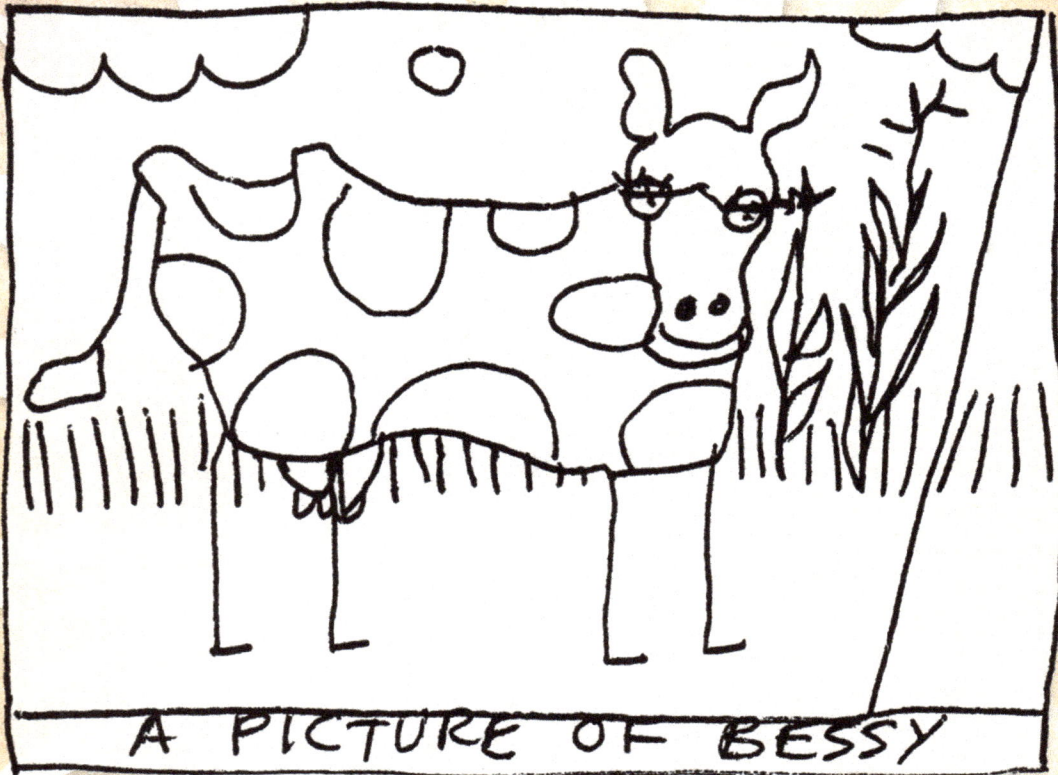

A PICTURE OF BESSY

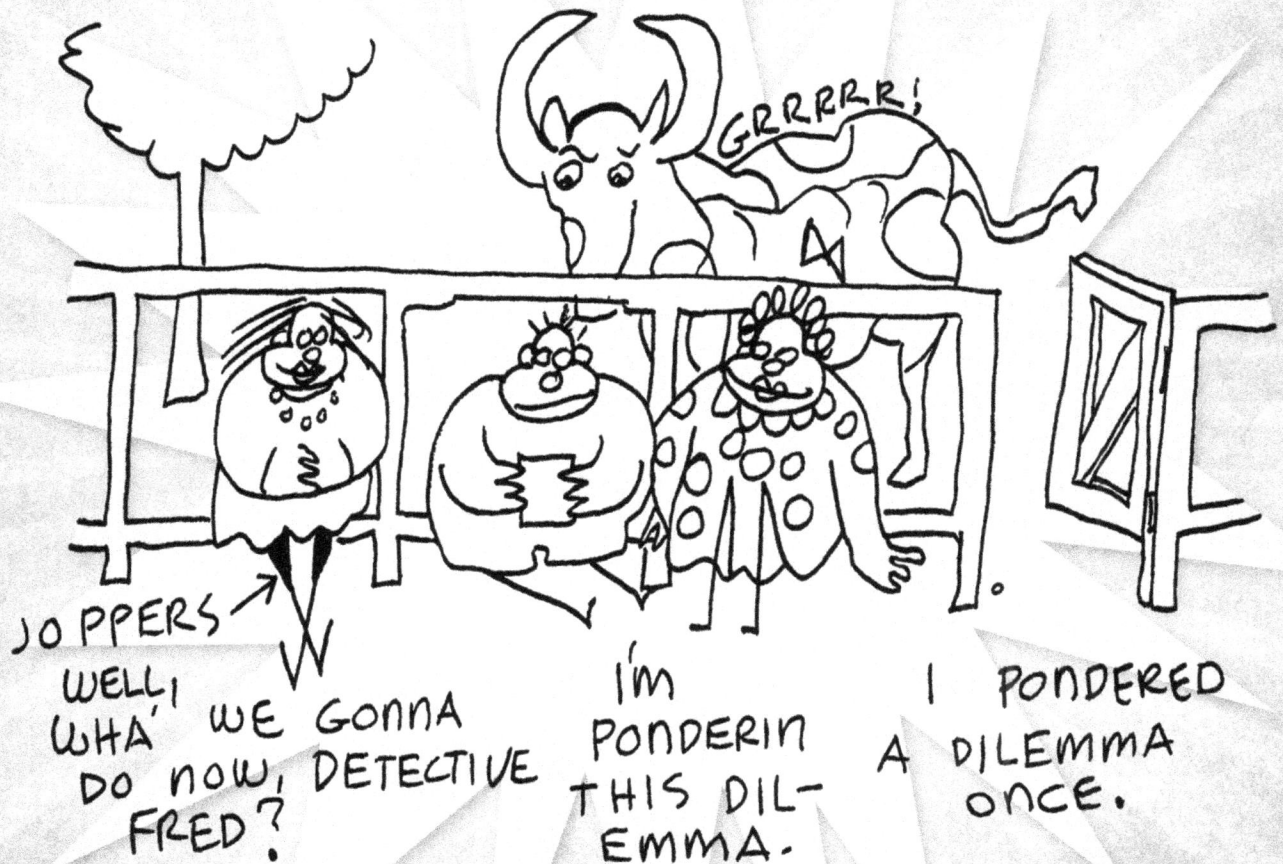

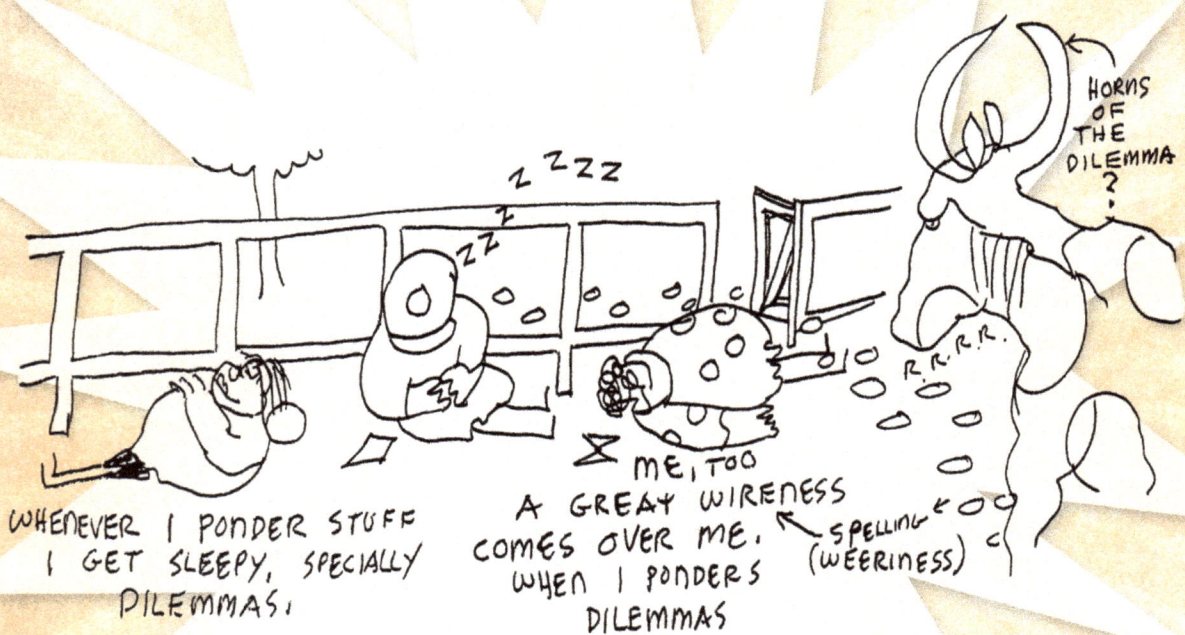

WHENEVER I PONDER STUFF
I GET SLEEPY, SPECIALLY
PILEMMAS.

Z ZZZ

ME, TOO
A GREAT WIRENESS
COMES OVER ME.
WHEN I PONDERS
DILEMMAS

SPELLING
(WEERINESS)

R.R.R.R.

HORNS
OF
THE
DILEMMA
?

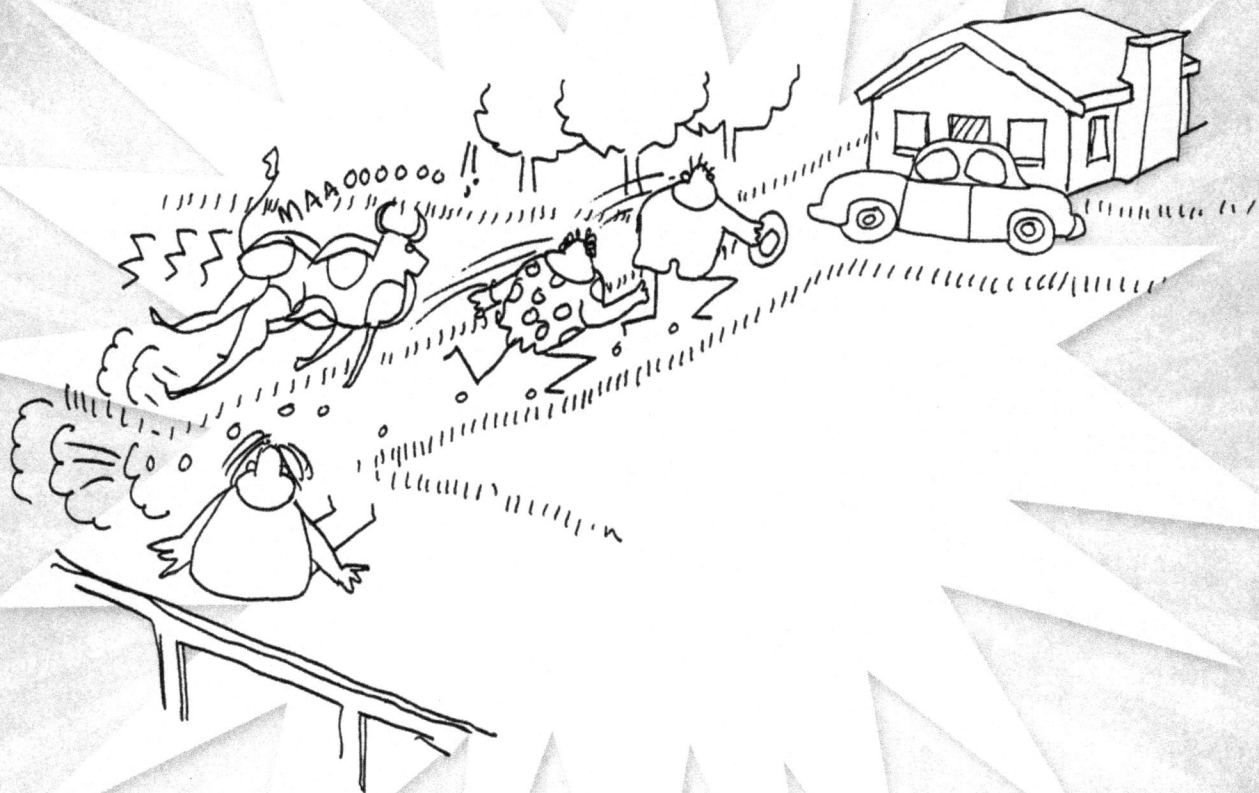

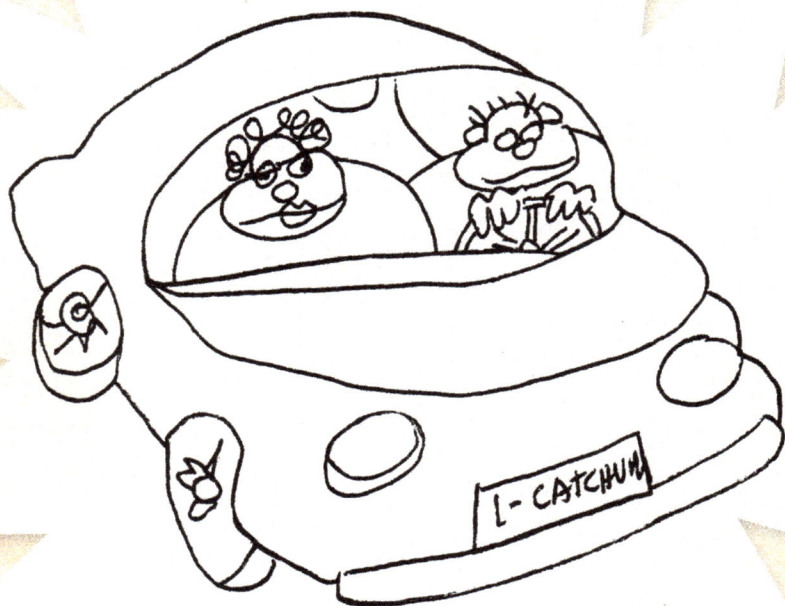

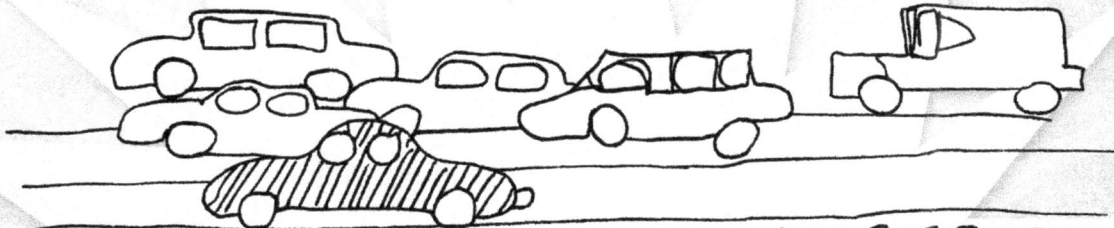

OK, FRED, WHERE WE GOIN?

WELL, FINALLY, AFTER 2 HRS YOU DECIDE TO TALK TO ME.

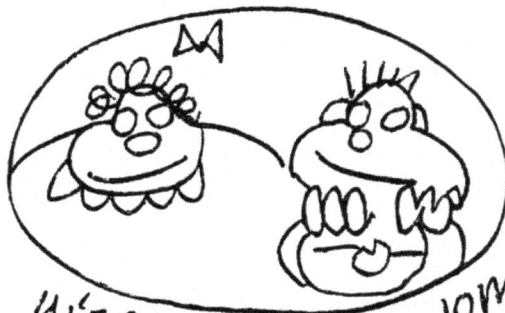

W'ERE GOIN HOME

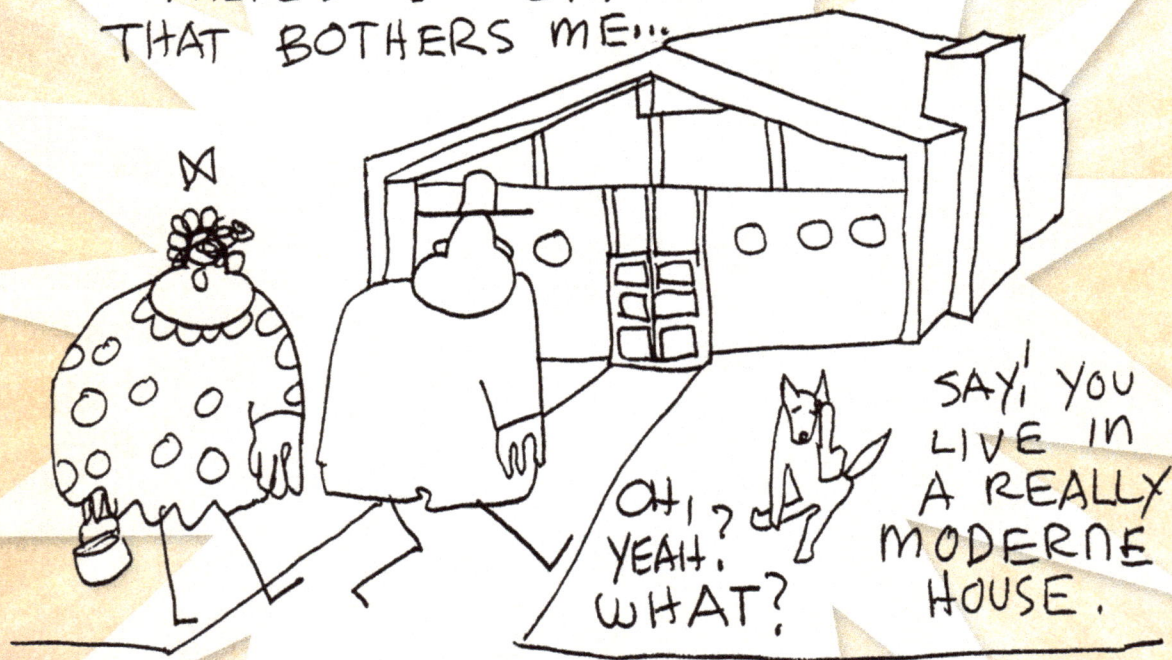

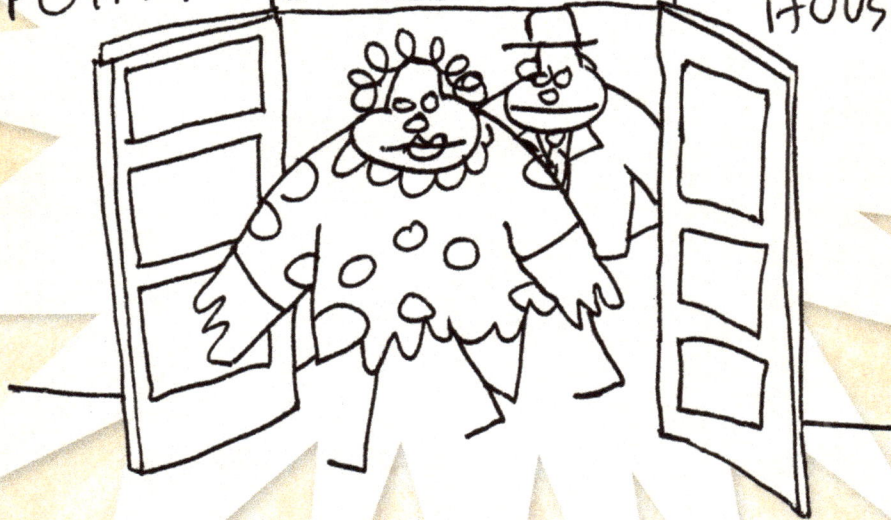

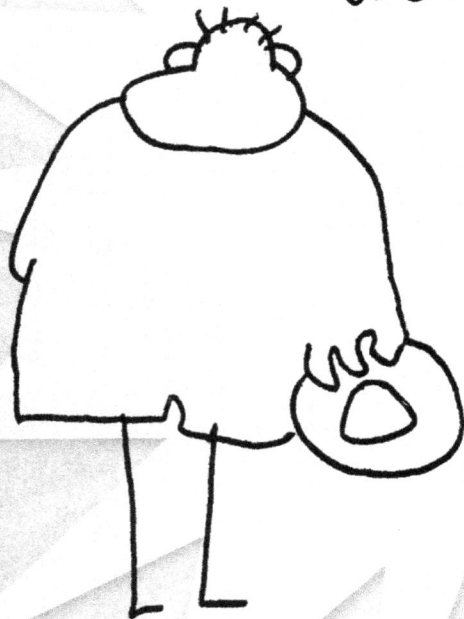
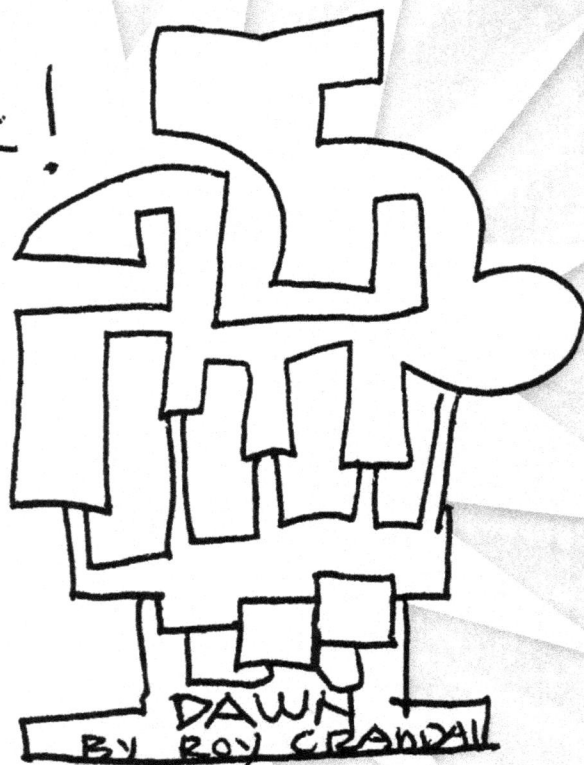

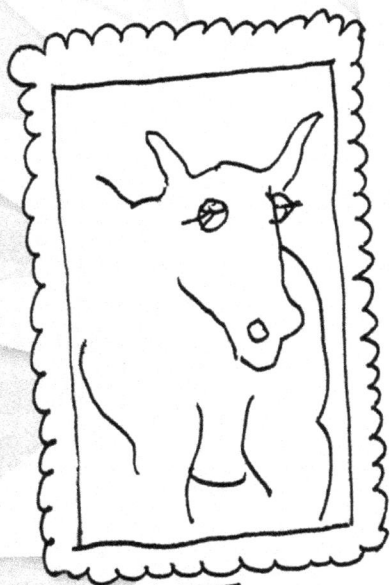

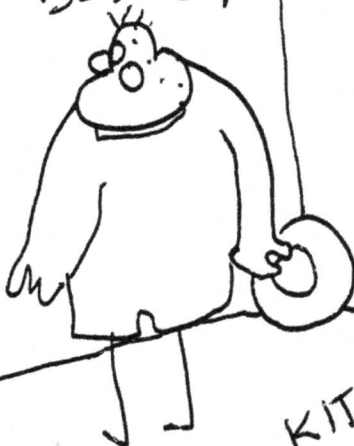

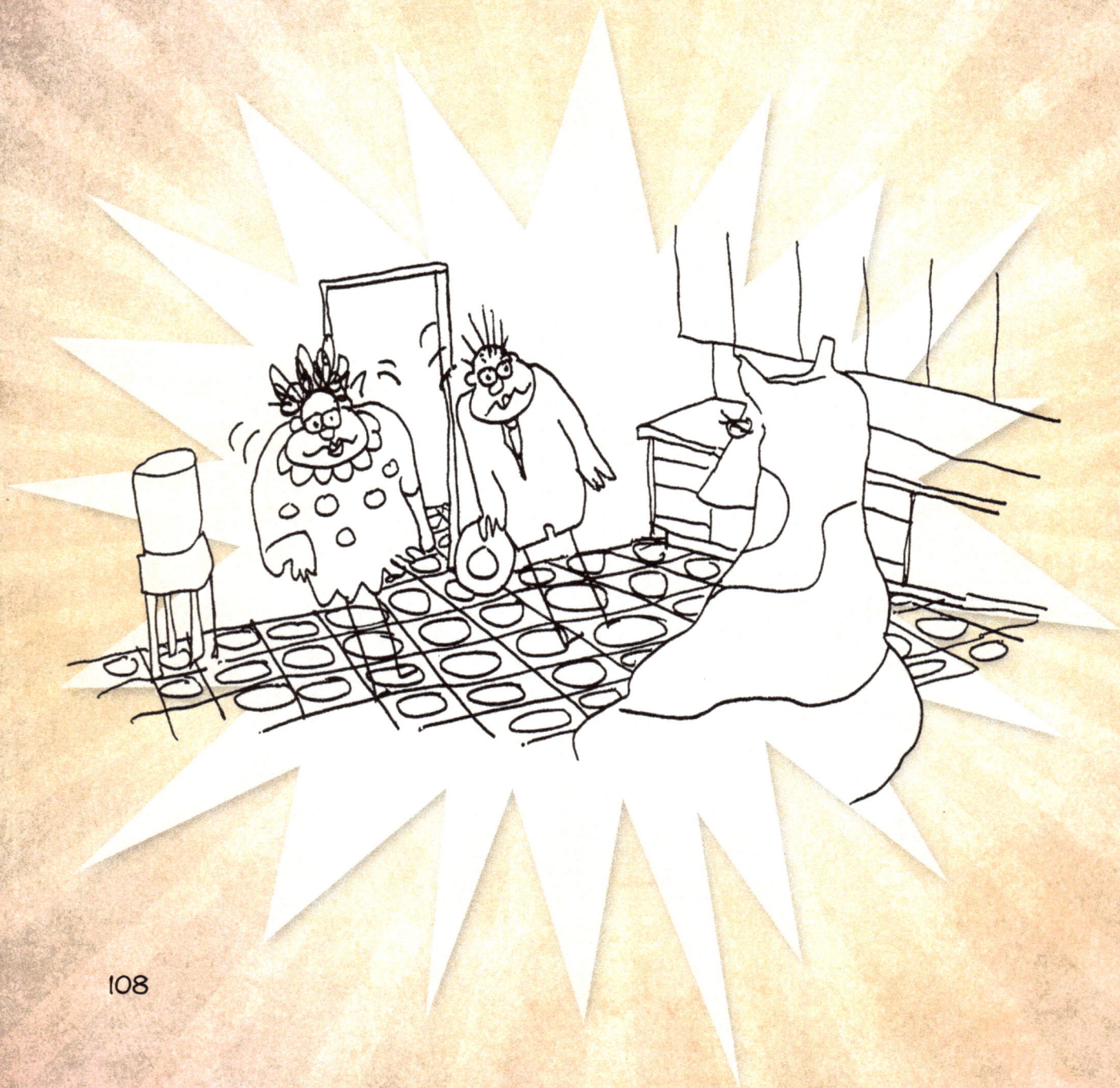

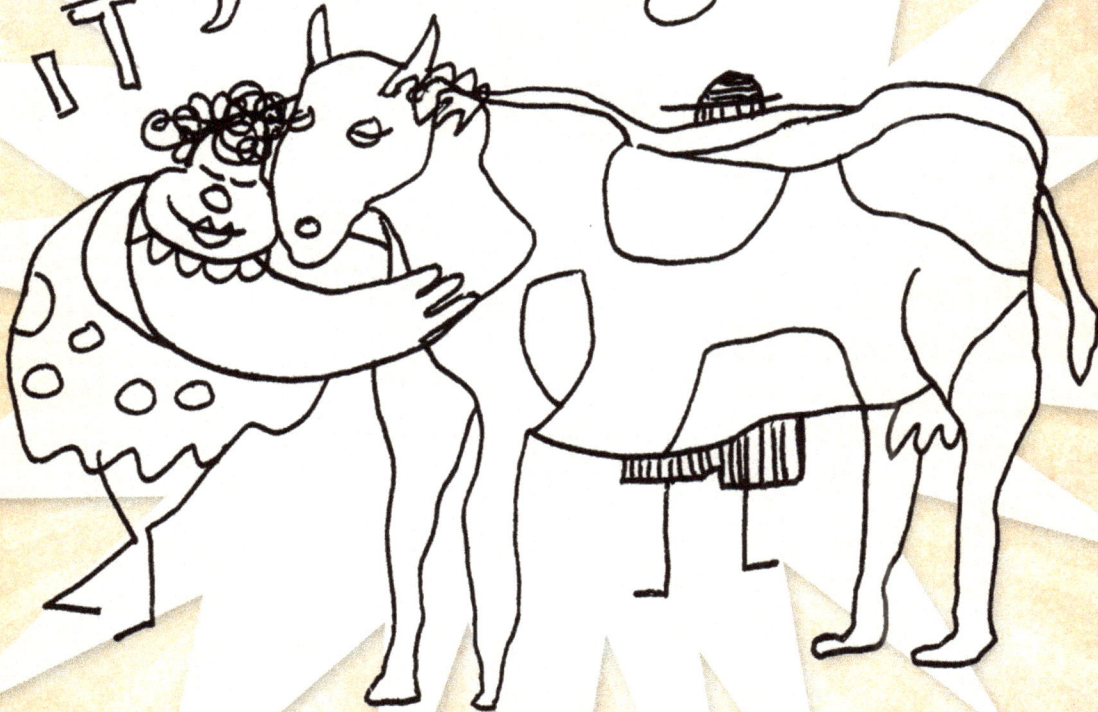

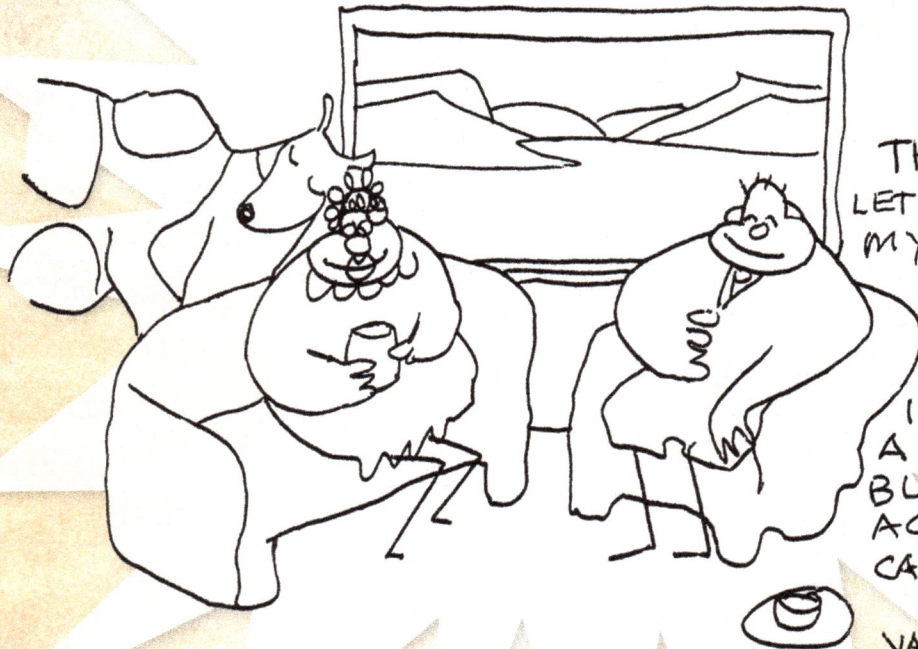

The End!

If you've got this far there is a serious chance your True mentality is showing. Better ditch this book before anyone notices. [You can sneak-read it later.]

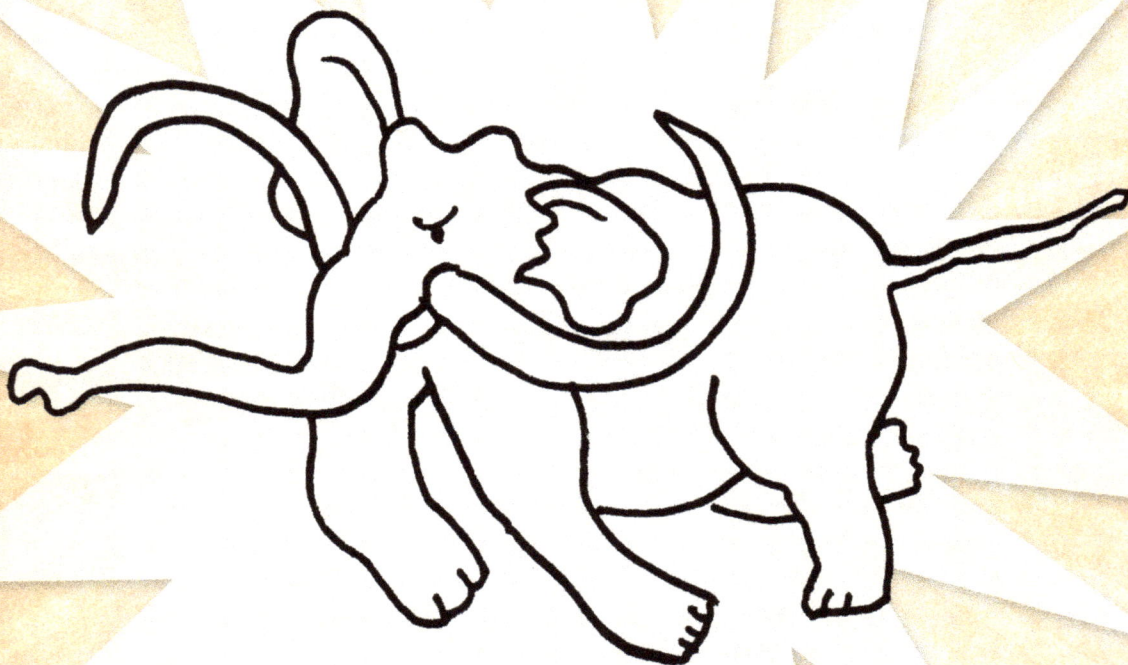

Other similar books by Doug Rucker

Cranthology
Where's the Cookies At?
A Book About Everyday Stuff
Book of Thoughts
Further Adventures
Maude
Tales of the Whorthwhile Dog
The Written Roy
Father Kokomo
Crandalicus

See Amazon for a complete list of books.
Roy Crandal is a pseudonym for Doug Rucker.